G000115885

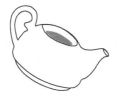

Praise for
Waking Up to Feeling

Alexandra Cabot has written a brave and beautiful memoir about her "expressive journey of intentional healing." Each of those four principle words matter. "Expressive" references the power of the expressive arts, including deep journaling and writing practices. "Journey" references Alexandra's life-long quest. "Intentional Healing" tells us this is a journey undertaken with the intention to move toward wholeness and the true self. I love this memoir for its freshness, its candor, and its open-hearted wonder at the precious lives we are given and what we each make of this gift.

Michael Lerner
Cofounder, Commonweal

Alexandra writes with a glorious freedom, braiding past and present with ease. She's a life-detective, hunting for meaning through a myriad of experiences, and bringing us along for the ride. As she moves naturally through memory and contemplation and back again, questions get asked, and some even answered. What has really worked? What has proved important? What does she know now that she didn't at the beginning? Certain solid truths emerge—never empty theories but lived realizations that make the difference between a life unexamined and one that keeps the lights up high. We visit childhood, adolescence, marriages, family, professions and friendships. Everything makes a difference. Everything is looked at closely in the most human of terms. And, most delightfully, you feel throughout that you are with one of your best friends, sitting in her comfortable living room, the fire going, and a tray of good coffee and snacks laid out before you. Keep this book by your side and you'll have a companion who doesn't claim to have everything figured out, but who will never stop looking for the meaning of it all.

Marta Szabo

Author of The Guru Looked Good and The Imposters

Waking Up to Feeling describes a journey from anguish and confusion to joy, from isolation to connection. Alexandra's story—written from the heart with gusto and courage—is one of transformation and healing, authentic and inspiring, and many will draw strength by finding their own reflection here. Alexandra has made a generous and valuable contribution to the literature of our times.

Barbara S. Kane, PhD
Psychoanalyst

In this beautifully written and intimate memoir, Alexandra untangles the life-long impact of love given and love withheld, battles with eczema and chronic illness, and the misguided decisions made over a lifetime. Specifically related to living with eczema, she gives voice to the completely life-altering disease that is still woefully misunderstood. She is by all accounts a woman warrior to have battled the incessant itch 24/7, along with the painful, red, inflamed skin, throughout her life. Woven throughout is a profound search for wholeness, especially as a mother. One of the powerful messages of this book is that it's never too late! It's never too late to come to know your own worthiness, to share your truth, to forgive mistakes, and live in compassion and empathy—often by simply noticing—with no analyzing or judgement. Lessons for all. It has led her to a spiritual acceptance that is honest and allows much grace for herself and others. Her crazy deep love for children, her children and grandchildren in particular, is a true wonder and inspiration. Her story is a gift to us all.

Julie Block
President & CEO
National Eczema Association

While still a toddler, Alexandra Cabot is abandoned by an alcoholic mother and soon afflicted with a chronic illness, akin to torture, that will recur throughout her life. Thus begins the author's life-long search for emotional and physical healing. Armed with a passionate and magnetic personality, and with generations of breeding that preclude self-pity, she builds and cares for a vast family that includes children, grandchildren, emotionally disabled siblings, and dozens of friends and employees. She also creates a school program to help underprivileged children who may suffer as she did as a child. An inspiring story of the power of giving and receiving love to heal emotional and physical trauma.

Nancy Hopkins
Amgen Inc Professor of Biology emerita
MIT

Waking Up to Feeling

An Expressive Journey of Intentional Healing

ALEXANDRA CABOT

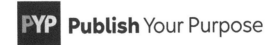

PYP Publish Your Purpose

For permission requests, write to the publisher, addressed "Attention: Permissions Coordinator," at the address below.

Publish Your Purpose
141 Weston Street, #155
Hartford, CT, 06141

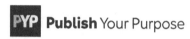

The opinions expressed by the Author are not necessarily those held by Publish Your Purpose.

Ordering Information: Quantity sales and special discounts are available on quantity purchases by corporations, associations, and others. For details, contact the publisher at hello@publishyourpurpose.com.

Edited by: Kris Jordan, August Li, Nancy Graham-Tillman
Cover design by: Cornelia Murariu
Typeset by: Medlar Publishing Solutions Pvt Ltd., India

Printed in the United States of America.
ISBN: 978-1-955985-68-0 (hardcover)
ISBN: 978-1-955985-67-3 (paperback)
ISBN: 978-1-955985-69-7 (ebook)

Library of Congress Control Number: 9781955985673

First edition, September 2022.

Publish Your Purpose is a hybrid publisher of non-fiction books. Our authors are thought leaders, experts in their fields, and visionaries paving the way to social change—from food security to anti-racism. We give underrepresented voices power and a stage to share their stories, speak their truth, and impact their communities. Do you have a book idea you would like us to consider publishing? Please visit PublishYourPurpose.com for more information.

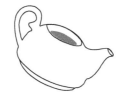

Dedication

I dedicate this memoir to my four children:
Sarah, Michael, Rachel, and Nathaniel.

Wisdom is a living stream, not an icon preserved in a museum. Only when we find the spring of wisdom in our own life can it flow to future generations.
—Thích Nhất Hạnh

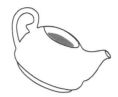

Table of Contents

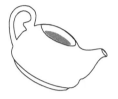

Preface

April 15, 2022

Sitting in the sunshine on my back porch, I have been gazing at a blossoming cherry tree in my backyard while talking on the phone to one of my closest friends. For over an hour now, we have been discussing how much we love our children and why I dedicated my book to them.

My life began to be entirely different once I was pregnant with my firstborn, Sarah. The realization that I was going to give birth and be able to raise a child changed my experience of being alive. I felt I had a purpose, and I was able to focus on being as good a mother as I could be. As you will read, much of my early life was quite unhappy, and although I talk a lot about those years, I want to make you aware of the transformation that came about when I had children.

One indication of my delight in looking forward to being a mother is that I started to read. Up until I was twenty-five years old, I had never really read for pleasure, but pending motherhood created a desire to find out about pregnancy and childbirth. I gradually became a voracious reader, and now that I can listen to audiobooks, I positively devour them with huge pleasure.

When Michael was born nineteen months after Sarah, I was exuberant to have a son. Then there was Rachel two and a half years later, and I was thrilled to have a second daughter. Next came Nathaniel, arriving two years after Rachel, giving me a complete family of two daughters and two sons. I felt jubilant.

I have a lovely memory of dancing with Jeremy, the father of all four of my children. We were at a Lincoln Nursery School party in Concord, Massachusetts. I had Nathaniel strapped to my front in a green carrier, and the three of us danced to "I Could Have Danced All Night." I felt blessed and was full of gratitude.

Each one of my children has turned out to be an adult that I admire, respect, and love with all my heart. Having just returned to my home in Rhinebeck, New York, after spending two weeks visiting three of these wonderful adults, I have seen that their lives are so full. I very much appreciate their efforts to keep in touch and am extremely fortunate to connect with them as often as I do. Happily, I also visited the fourth one recently, and here is what I consider a miracle: each one of these offspring is an exceptionally sensitive, caring, and superb parent! I am passionately interested in parenting, and to have the privilege of watching them raise their children is a major blessing of my life. I pray they will understand that I needed to write my story as a way of healing my childhood.

This past winter I revised a portrait interview that I did last September, which includes an enormous number of photographs of my children and grandchildren as well as other family and friends. A one-hour video was created from six hours of conversation with David Patrick Adams up in Northfield, Vermont, and his wife, Maria Lucia Ferreira, edited it.

My reason for writing this memoir and doing a portrait interview was not as much to be a good ancestor as it was to view my own life with more compassion. Now that this goal has been accomplished, I see better why I have made some of the mistakes I have made and am more forgiving than before.

My ability to express my experience has been transformative. As I now see it, no matter how this book is received, I benefit. So, it is with humility that I now hope it may be of some help to someone else. My gratitude to each of my four children is as profound as my deep love.

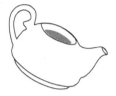

Acknowledgments

The spiritual life is about becoming more at home in your own skin.

—Parker J. Palmer

Two years ago, just before the pandemic, I signed up for a workshop in New York City (NYC) called "Fearless Communicators." The founder, Eduardo Pincer, took us out to dinner the first evening, where I sat next to a woman I had never met before named Jenn Grace. When she told me she helped people write their stories, I was intrigued. I began working with Jenn a few weeks later, and it is because of her that I have been able to complete this memoir.

The process of writing has brought me a new awareness of being comfortable in my skin. There will still be outbreaks of eczema, but I will greet them as a signal for me to slow down and take care of my own inner being.

The above quote from Parker J. Palmer intrigues me because my eczema is healed at the time of this writing. I have been following Grand Master Lu's Chinese medical Qigong practices for nearly two years now, and I choose to believe that this, in part, has led to my skin clearing. The combination of writing, reading, and practicing Qigong has worked for me.

I believe we all have to find our own way, but I could not have done it without the following people, to whom I give my deepest gratitude: Jenn Grace, founder and CEO of Publish your Purpose Press; Kris Jordan, writing coach; Winifred Marion, Qigong practitioner; Marta Szabo, founder and co-director of Authentic Writing Workshops; Paula Throckmorten, meditation leader; Barbara Kane, psychoanalyst; and Charles Castle.

I know I have been exceedingly fortunate for so many people in my life, and I want to express my deep appreciation to my longtime Spence School friends, my Florida friends, and my Rhinebeck friends. I also wish to thank my companion, who has chosen the pseudonym Monica. Without all of you, I never could have completed this book.

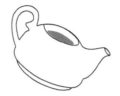

Introduction

I decided to see if writing, which I have found therapeutic, might help me like myself more. Having written this book, I now see it has done that. I have more compassion for my struggles, especially regarding my response to the time of COVID-19. One reason for this is because my life is blurry as I look back. Perhaps you will understand this better as you read on. Hopefully, this book will at least show how one woman of seventy-five years looks at her life, both now and before COVID.

For many decades I have wanted to give my life meaning and share my experiences, so I have taken numerous writing workshops and classes and just finished two that I have enjoyed during this pandemic. It is very strange to be getting close to eighty and not feel old at all, and my heartfelt desire is to connect with each of my grandchildren. I pray I can complete this memoir and that my grandchildren will feel they know their Nonnie better and can better appreciate her quirks after hearing of her struggles.

I want this memoir to focus on my healing. I want to question whether I unconsciously sought healing for a long time before I intentionally sought it. When I tell you even a little about myself, it will become pretty obvious that I have been enormously privileged. So, right away, I need to state that I am grateful for all that I have been able to pursue, including psychotherapy, workshops, and integrative medical treatments.

Today, I have a house and home I love here in the Hudson River valley in the village of Rhinebeck, New York. I have lovely neighbors and even a live-in caregiving companion, Monica. She comes from St. Lucia and is a truly remarkable woman. Her deep faith in God has rubbed off on me. She simply embodies kindness and gives me the motherly loving attention I have wanted my entire life. I am aware that I would not be in the good health I am finally experiencing if it were not for Monica.

I also have four wonderful children and ten beautiful grandchildren and am living without the Rolodex of anxieties that once ran my life. I wake up looking forward to each day and seem to always be busy enough, but I no longer rush through each day. I can announce to you that I feel content, except for when something triggers me.

Introduction

My struggles with lifelong eczema, gut issues, and learning disabilities have resulted in my feeling intense self-consciousness. Now that I am learning how my past has influenced my experience of living, I have realized that I was unable to allow my emotions to flow. I am finding new perspectives, especially in the areas of energy healing, therapeutic writing, and community connectedness, and am enjoying the new rituals I have adopted that help me understand myself more deeply. These include Healing Circles, pendulums, Qigong, journal writing, reading, listening to audiobooks, and watching videos. The Healing Circles are helping me learn to trust silence, and Qigong is helping me become disciplined and move my energy. Journal writing has proven to be therapeutic and gives structure to my day, and watching videos and reading have helped me learn more about how I can heal from trauma. Gradually, I am becoming able to alter my tendency to put pleasing others ahead of my own needs. I am less impulsive now that I see how frequently I want to leap to action.

I am scheduling fewer people into my days, which allows for space and peaceful rest in between my activities. This is coinciding with my awareness of physical comfort and emotional ease. For instance, when I notice that I am not bothered by leg cramps while lying in bed, I delight in the sensation of stretching and finding a cool spot on the sheets for my feet, realize my good fortune, and send a prayer for others who are suffering in so many ways.

I have also become aware of my need to be busy and constantly please people. The more I learn about myself, relationships, and the world, the more comfortable I become. I am intrigued by what I have been drawn to and have come to believe that nothing in my life experience has been wasted. Everything seems to come full circle; everything is indeed connected. And I am healing.

The past few weeks, I have gotten away from my routine, and it has been really hard to reestablish it. I have just had a day that has put me in a very low mood, and that makes me feel vulnerable and sad. So, it is not as though I have it all together at all, and I think no one really has it figured out—at least, I haven't met anyone who does. We can lean on our friends if we are fortunate and have them. Some people rely on other sources of comfort, but for me, friends are the most reliable. They remind me that I am loveable. If we can remember that we have some goodness inside, that helps a lot.

I was told that in Africa when a person is suffering a setback or an illness, the person's tribe and family surround them and remind them of their goodness. This appeals to me, as I think we who can reach out to others manage to create a similar Healing Circle. Overall, I have found that if we see ourselves as all connected, we are kinder and more empathetic, and that is needed today.

Introduction

I am using this pandemic as my timeline; it is providing me with the framework for my story. Even this morning as I write this, I am looking pathetic with a red rash on my face and my eyes all puffy. They itch and so do my hands. The flare-up of my skin is a time for me to look at the root cause. And you may not be surprised to hear my conclusion that I will never really understand the mixture of reasons why my body and psyche have this dance.

The book you are about to read is about my experience of struggling and searching for answers. I want to emphasize how each of us is trying to get our needs met. Some of us are more capable of reaching out for solutions than others, especially right now in the summer of 2021 when we are facing a series of so many crises that people are using the term "polycrisis." May we all pray that this, too, will pass. Individually, we may have little ability to change the course of our future, yet, if we are among the fortunate, we are still able to maneuver our well-being. I have no answers here, this is just another example of a human struggle we must endure and a reminder to enjoy the mystery of life.

It is also important to know that this memoir includes vignettes that follow themes more than chronological order. Some names have been changed to protect the personal identity of those I am referencing. I have also included some of my favorite quotes and have compiled some of my favorite resources, many of which

I cite throughout the book. I hope they bring you as much delight as they have me.

This channeled quote from Patrick S. Wolfe as referenced by David Spangler has become my inspiration and mantra and opens the story quite well:

> May all who can, open to the qualities of fiery hope, peace, joy, and love, and to the potential and energy of the new civilization unfolding around us. May love, not fear, hope, not despair, joy, not distress, compassion, not anger or hate, enfold each of us in safety, protection, and courage. May we have the will to do what is available to us to bring the new civilization into being. May my strength, my calm, my courage, my joy, my love, empower at least one other person to join in this enterprise and become a source of vision and new life.[1]

---

1. David Spangler, "David's Desk 173 Climate Crisis," Lorian, October 1, 2021, https://lorian.org/community/2021/9/27/davids-desk-173-climate-crisis.

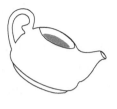

CHAPTER 1

Beginning My Search for Healing

You wear a mask for so long, you forget who you were beneath it.

—Alan Moore, *V for Vendetta*

I am sitting upstairs in my New York home during a snowstorm. I have only two commitments today: my weekly Zoom call with "Rhinebeck at Home" at 4:00 p.m. and my daily meditation call, also on Zoom. The meditation is led by Paula, a friend of my younger daughter's. During the meditation, I often fall asleep or at least go to some other realm. My mind goes somewhere where I become invariably startled when I hear Paula's gentle voice after a few minutes of silence.

While Paula guides us in her informal meditation, I am sometimes able to follow her and often I am not, but I try to never miss this delicious ending to my day.

During this pandemic year, I am writing a memoir in which I am choosing not to look at my life's many chapters with the intention of taking them all apart. I have spent most decades of my life examining and trying to understand why things have happened as they have. Now I am in a new place and have what I hope is a fresh perspective. With less analyzing and more noticing, I have come to believe that none of my life has been wasted and have found myself with more questions and curiosity than answers.

This morning I once again correctly guessed the time I would wake up within three minutes—3:50 a.m.! I have a wall clock in my bathroom, so I play this game several times a night. It gives me a little dab of pleasure when my guess is within five minutes of the actual time.

After I put on my cozy, blue bathrobe and tan, sheepskin-lined slippers, I put the electric kettle on in the kitchen and quietly empty the dishwasher. Meanwhile, I use the instant hot water to heat up the teapot and my mug, get a tray ready to take into the living room, light a candle, click the remote to turn on the gas fire, and then turn on the lamps.

I fix the tea as I like it, with a bit of oat milk and a teaspoon of honey, and settle in for my two daily readings before I write in my journal. This takes about half an hour. I read until about 6:30 a.m., then I take my shower, get dressed, and bring my phone upstairs to do my Qigong with Master Lu showing me his "Dragon's Way" practice via DVD. I have been doing these exercises every day for the last six months. While I move all those complicated meridians, I am also exercising to have more energy or chi. I used to listen to an Audible book on my cell phone while I did The Dragon's Way, but I realized that what I am trying to strengthen is my ability to focus. So now I just do the exercises without listening to something else. Some days I follow this with Dr. Zach Bush's "The Four Minute Workout," and occasionally I will remember to fit in two more repetitions of this workout later in the day.

So here I am, a woman who could never keep a schedule, wanting structure so badly that I have created an actual routine, and I think it is keeping me sane. I almost never rush any more. No wonder life has become a pleasure. But it has not always been that way.

❋ ❀ ❋ ❀ ❋

The search for healing has led me to a deepening faith. My lifelong struggle with eczema has led to a curiosity about what it may be telling me. What is so hard is that I have more questions than answers. My personal dynamics and history and this time away from others is causing me to reflect on many questions that come to my mind. What I now see as my purpose is to attempt to become a more loving person.

Through learning about the connections between early childhood trauma and adult disease, I am gradually discovering a way to view my struggle with more compassion and hopefully understanding. I am seeing that maybe my eczema is a metaphor. Perhaps my little infant Self needed to express the rage she felt.

My mother gave birth to me in the Boston Lying-in Hospital on December 22, 1943. I was in the room that day when Mummy told Daddy she wanted a divorce. My father had been away in the navy in the Mediterranean for nine months, and during that time Mummy had fallen in love with a senior partner in the law firm that my father had been in. Mummy probably did not say that she had become an alcoholic, even before the time I was conceived. She may not have been able to admit this addiction. She was hospitalized several times in psychiatric hospitals but never would attend Alcoholics Anonymous meetings.

My first outbreak of severe eczema came when I was two months old, riding overnight on a train with my grandmother who had never taken care of me before. I had a nanny, but she was left behind. When my mother and her brother met the train in Florida, they rushed me to the emergency room in the local hospital where the doctor diagnosed my skin rash as atopic dermatitis.

I never lived under the same roof with both my parents, and when I was two years old, I was moved to New York City to live with my father, along with my three older brothers. This was after Mummy relinquished custody of all four of us.

In 1946, after three months in that new home on Park Avenue in Manhattan, I was put into the hospital. I had pulled out most of my hair, and there were open sores all over my face and body. I was admitted with pneumonia, pleurisy, and severe eczema. I was there in New York Hospital for a month. I remember this hospitalization partly because of the pain, but even more because Anna Lundgren, our family cook, came to bring me a present on my third birthday. When Anna saw that the nurse had tied my hands to the bed so I could not scratch, she cried. After the ties were loosened, I was able to open the birthday present. It was a tea set, and I was enchanted by it. I still recall Anna wiping away her tears and smiling.

The next hospitalization was in 1953. This time I was admitted into the Beth Israel Hospital in Boston under the care of an extraordinary dermatologist, Dr. Richard Hoffman, who cared for me for the four weeks I was there. It was the happiest month of my childhood because I was finally getting the attention I craved. I was a problem in fifth grade that year at the Spence School, a private all-girls school, and I sought attention by acting out. I taught some of my classmates how to shoplift. Other friends knew better than to follow through with it, and they still cared for me.

I still claim close friendships with five of these Spence pals. Isn't it remarkable that at age seventy-seven I still have friends from that fifth-grade class? It is probably no surprise that I became a social worker after studying family therapy and realizing that children act out for a reason. Many decades later, I enjoyed working in Boston for the Massachusetts Society for the Prevention of Cruelty to Children.

Friendship is one thing I can vouch for in this life. I am less sure about everything else, but the support and love friends have given me are why I am still here, curious, and amazingly more content than before the pandemic.

* * * * *

I wrote a letter to Rumi, the writer of the poem "The Guest House," and told him that I have spent decades racing through my life. I would cram as much activity into each day as I could, and that resulted in my feeling I had done something. But now that such rushing is not rewarded or really possible, I still want a sense of accomplishment and am an absolute lunatic about keeping my house tidy. I did not used to care that much, but if my house is a mess, I feel a mess inside my head. Hence, I have learned to return things to a place I can find them again.

The other emotion that has come up repeatedly is deep sadness. When I am reminded of all the suffering people in the world, I feel such helplessness and sorrow beyond words. Yet what can I learn from this? I feel that this bewildering time is actually teaching us to become introspective and discover our inner Selves. I choose to call this bewildering time "an evolution of consciousness." I am becoming more confident. I realize that I need to consider my behavior and be courteous, but I can come closer to thinking for myself. The realization that we choose which truth to believe is profoundly unsettling. I have my identity wrapped around what I have come to believe, and yet I realize that this, too, I must relinquish. I may well be wrong.

I am also learning to savor relationships and be less dependent on outside validation. Actually, writing this makes me smile because one of the new things I use in my life is a pendulum, and I now depend a lot on what the pendulum says. Anger and sadness have brought me clearer knowledge of who I am, what I can change, and what I cannot.

To my delight, I have become more aware of the wonders of nature. I heard a bird's song last week and was ecstatic. Spring really will come and at its own pace. I am more conscious of how our paces differ and am becoming a tiny bit more patient. I take walks alone and like the solitude and am tasting food with more appreciation. Yesterday, when we were both in the kitchen while she listened to me on the phone with AppleCare, Monica told me that I was a very patient woman!

I just put the large coffee-table-sized book called *Dolly* down in the kitchen for Monica who loves Dolly Parton's music as much as I do. Monica is making chicken stock from all the bones she has collected in the freezer in a plastic bag. We will have chicken soup for lunch today. It is totally miraculous for me to be so absorbed all by myself these days.

※　❋　※　❋　※

When I first met Monica, I was struck by how she radiated a sense of comfort. "Those pastries look amazing!" Monica said, and I agreed. The waitress poured her a cup of coffee and set down a cup and tea selections for me. The other two friends at the table ordered their favorite drinks while we looked over the menu of homemade soups, sandwiches, and wonderful breakfast choices.

"The avocado toast sounds good too," Monica added. "And it's healthier for me."

"It really is delicious here. You can't go wrong with any choice, though," I added, dipping my tea bag in the hot water.

Monica is about my height, 5'6", is sixty-five years old, and has a slightly stocky build. She is reserved and introverted. At our first meeting, she did not ask questions but seemed relaxed. I looked at her face and saw soft, dark brown eyes. She seemed secure with who she is and reminded me of that on our first day of sharing cinnamon buns. Our conversation was easy, as she shared about her interest in politics, something she was interested in even as a little girl in St. Lucia. I could not care less about politics, but we both agreed the healthy avocado toast was a great choice. Monica and I were meeting as a mutual interview, in a sense. She was looking for a new living situation, and I was considering a companion to help me around the house.

After the meal, I showed Monica around my newly remodeled home. The tour included what would be her room and private bathroom. I explained how I felt she could help and what I was able to pay her. Today it is amazing to realize how quickly we agreed to a trial arrangement: if, after three months, either of us did not like living together, we would stop with no hard feelings. I am impulsive, and I liked this woman, particularly the fact that she already knew Rhinebeck and wanted to be near the village because she does not drive.

My fifty-year-old daughter was rather startled when I told her I was considering hiring a companion. "But Mom, you aren't sick!" she challenged.

"Honey," I told her, "I know that when you were a child, you received unconditional love from me. I haven't had that, and for me, this feels like the time I start to get some of that for myself."

Tears welled up in her eyes, and she seemed to be persuaded. Monica has been helping me for three years now.

When I was young, Mummy used to tell me, "I never wanted you." I had three older brothers and she would add that she only wanted the oldest of my brothers. My father loved us as best he could, but it was a pretty tough situation. I was told my second oldest brother, Michael, had been dropped as a baby by my mother. He required surgery to have a part of his brain removed and had Jacksonian epilepsy as a result. It was common for him to have grand mal seizures while we were growing up. I don't remember how often he had them, but they were very scary. Meanwhile, I was covered with severe eczema and was nearly bald. I spent my childhood shuffling between visiting my mother and stepfather in Beverly Farms, Massachusetts, during the summers and New York City the rest of the year.

Two of my brothers teased me incessantly. The brain-damaged one threw me down the stairs one time when he was angry. He said it was because I got too many phone calls. My father was not a disciplinarian, and my brothers were not reprimanded for tickling me unmercifully or hiding behind doors and frightening me at night. My father remarried when I was six, and he and my stepmother went on to have four more children. I was the youngest of the first litter and the eldest of the second. My stepmother called me the "lynchpin" of the family. All I wanted was to be taken care of and not criticized for being "overly sensitive," "too honest," or "too much of a live wire." My placement in the family did allow me to care for my younger siblings, though, and created a strong desire to have my own children one day.

I had not realized that the words I shared with my daughter were revealing such a yearning for unconditional love, or that deep down inside, my spirit knew Monica would meet that need. I later told a close friend about the arrangement with Monica.

"How will you introduce her to people?" she inquired.

I thought for a moment. "I guess I'll just say, 'I'd like you to meet my friend Monica.'"

My friend objected, "You can't call her your friend, because I am your friend; you can't have someone who works for you be a friend."

I disagreed, and we let it drop without resolution. I knew that if Monica and I liked one another, we would become friends whether money was exchanged or not. Looking at how antithetical our backgrounds are, one would think friendship unlikely, however. Monica's background is one of poverty in St. Lucia. When she was little, there were times when having meat was not possible, and she remembers fondly her father's vegetable garden that was essential for the family's sustenance. The children knew to respect their parents, and the result of her upbringing has left the siblings close and caring deeply for one another. She is the oldest of ten children, and she calls them in St. Lucia every night. She always talks with her mother as well.

Monica had a British school education and then taught for two years in St. Lucia. When she came to New York City, she received training as a caregiver and is now a home health aide. She worked as a cleaning person, but mostly she has been an aide for people who are dying in their homes. She likes her work and always goes home for at least a month each year to be with her family in St. Lucia.

I, on the other hand, had all the advantages of a fine education and all the things one associates with wealth. Clearly, I am a woman who has benefited from white privilege all my life. I had a cook preparing meals in both my mother's and father's homes. I also had a mother who was very proud of her ex-husband's lineage. She told me, "You are the direct descendant of Governor John Winthrop, who founded Harvard College as well as started the Massachusetts Bay Colony. You are the eleventh generation, and that makes you an American aristocrat."

However, I have also been textured by my life. The pain of living with severe eczema created decades of yearning for relief from that physical agony. While my family was large, it was very fractured, both from disease and divorce.

I know that the difference in Monica's and my backgrounds is startling. We come, in effect, from opposite ends of the class structure. She and I would never have met if she were not my employee. But there is something else between us that, at least in my mind, has allowed me to transcend the base economic realities.

Monica was raised by parents who were devout in the Catholic faith. She and her siblings are close and have their own variations of that religion. What Monica is confident of is that God is in charge. She relies on the Bible for her explanations and gently reminds me that all my books that I quote from are often saying what is right there in the Bible.

Two of my friends who never volunteer a hug toward me always go over to Monica when they come in and give her a hug. I think it is their desire to make Monica feel welcome in our predominantly white community. Something about Monica shows on the outside what a caring and dear person she is inside. A friend who only met Monica once remarked, "She is a real treasure, Alexandra."

I don't need to be told about every single thing that Monica does; I see it every day and am so grateful for it, and she knows it. I benefit in many ways from her presence. We chuckle over things. We are able to speak up about what works and what does not. The best adjustment came about when Monica told me she likes to do things at her own pace. She likes to take her time and do things carefully, and I move fast and am still impulsive. "We are all different, Alexandra," she reminded me one day early on in our relationship. "Our differences are okay; no reason for fear." On my seventy-eighth birthday, Monica's 7:30 a.m. call from St. Lucia was my first greeting. She and her sisters all sang "Happy Birthday" to me.

Happily, we now have a sort of rhythm that works very well. One morning before the pandemic, I came into the kitchen as Monica was making her coffee. I told her about an idea I had: "What do you think of the possibility of me coming down to spend January next year in St. Lucia? I'd love to meet your family."

"Alexandra, I just had exactly that idea myself! My sister can give you a house to stay in."

"Oh no, Monica, you are down there to be with your family. I will stay in a hotel not too far away."

A few minutes later, we were sitting on our stools in the kitchen. Monica said, "That idea, you know, that was our Guides at work!"

She chuckled and I smiled. A year ago, I did not believe in "Guides" or "Angels," but I have woken up to the possibility. I now believe more the way Monica does. I believe there is a loving energy we call God. The easiest indication is watching nature and being in awe of its complexity and mystery. Maybe there is some reason for the pandemic that we cannot know. Maybe we are being changed and good will eventually come of it.

If I am judged negatively for saying something as naive and simplistic as this, I no longer care. I am choosing to believe that we are going through an evolution of consciousness that we are unable to alter. As Monica keeps saying, "God is in charge. We need to trust that He will use all things to make our world better."

Most startling to me lately is my sense of well-being. I have been told that healing is multilayered, and I have benefited from acupuncture, supplements, massage, and other treatments. My thoughts turn to Monica and the emotional climate she has created by her very presence. Never before have I been with someone who gives to me with no judgment. Is it possible that there really are no accidents? This idea once seemed crazy, but not anymore. The fact that I have been able to travel and receive expert medical and psychological help has been beneficial, for sure. But I wonder if having Monica here has been the most healing of all the treatments I have sought.

My experience is that I can now accept and, yes, maybe even love myself in a way that was not possible before Monica came to live with me. How she is able to give that unconditional love remains a mystery. She says it is part of God's plan and "Yes, it is a mystery, but God is in charge."

So my question is, can we be friends even if money is exchanged? Or do we say we are "*Anam Cara*" or "Soul Friends" and let that be good enough?

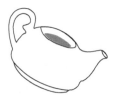

CHAPTER 2

Looking Back

Teaching is humbling. I know I have more
to learn, particularly around the blind spots
of my own privilege.

—Oren Jay Sofer

Today is my oldest child's fifty-second birthday. Her name is Sarah, and it is fun for me to look back on that morning of March 5th, 1969. At 1:00 a.m., I felt my very first contraction, but I did not wake my husband. I was well-read in all the natural childbirth literature, so I knew the birth of this baby was many hours away from my going to Lenox Hill Hospital.

As it happened, I had contractions all through that day and even persuaded my friend Jenny accompany me to a movie. She and I were teaching that year at the

Dalton School in NYC, and she was also pregnant but not due for another two months.

I was so excited to be having a baby. It felt like "at long last," as I had wanted a baby nine months after our honeymoon. But it took three years for me to get pregnant, and I am not a patient person. Sarah's father and I had moved from up near Columbia University to directly across 77th Street so my doctor could deliver this baby at Lenox Hill Hospital.

By dinnertime these contractions were getting really strong. I was ecstatic when Dr. Nash finally suggested I could come across the street and meet him up on the maternity floor. In the elevator of our building, I had another powerful contraction but managed not to cry out, as I could see the elevator man looked pretty frightened.

When we came through the side entrance, I was relieved to be given a wheelchair. Staff took me up to the maternity floor and said goodbye to my husband, who was told to go on home and that Dr. Nash would give him a call when it was all over. Then there were several hours of waiting. My back pain became unbearable, but I just cried; I did not scream. My doctor finally told me I would have to be given anesthesia because my baby was "sunny-side up." He said he needed to turn the baby around and then it would go quickly.

I remember feeling relieved but also sad. I had so wanted to watch my baby arrive, but such excruciating pain made me compliant and I gave no resistance. I heard yelling from another mother in labor, and the next thing I knew I was in the recovery room. Had I had a boy or a girl? When a nurse told me I had a baby girl, I cried with delight.

While I was in my hospital room, I got a call from a friend of my parents, Mrs. Wheelock. She was not someone I felt close to at all, but my husband had dutifully called my parents and his to tell them of our little baby Sarah's birth, and Mummy had called Mrs. Wheelock. She called to say how sorry she was to hear that I had had a girl but wanted to congratulate me anyway! I was appalled and speechless.

Mrs. Wheelock's daughter, who was just a little younger than me, bonded with me over having three older brothers and being the only girl. Her brother, same age as me, hung himself when we were eighteen. That information was a phone call I remember well because I got the news on a hall telephone at Briarcliff College. It was my first experience of knowing someone who ended their life on purpose.

That morning, my pediatrician, Dr. Nauss, entered the room with the cart that held Sarah. I leaped out of the bed and came over to watch him gently unfold the blanket so I could gaze at my daughter for the first time.

"Isn't she beautiful, Alexandra?" I was speechless as I looked at this enchanting newborn. She had black hair that stood straight up and exquisite dark brown eyes that looked right at me. When I realized that Dr. Nauss was counting her toes I said, "I'm sorry Doctor, I wasn't paying attention. Is she missing a finger, or is it a toe?"

He laughed and said, "Oh no, I was just showing you how perfect she is."

❋ ❋ ❋ ❋ ❋

Today I am really happy. What makes for this mood of excitement and discovery? I have just listened to Dr. Gabor Maté give a lecture that helped me understand myself. I think it must be the same feeling that Monica feels when she nears the end of one of her very difficult one-thousand-piece jigsaw puzzles.

I have finally seen what impact my mother's life had on me, and I don't know where to start. On the day I was born, December 22, 1943, my father came back from serving on a destroyer in the Mediterranean. In the hospital, Mummy told Daddy she wanted a divorce. I never asked my father anything about this scene, and I wonder why I didn't.

After my daddy died in 1980, my stepmother gave me the letters that Daddy had saved. It was then that I read the one from Mummy, written when I was still an infant. The letter gave my father custody of all four of their children. She said she felt so guilty she wanted him to raise me and my three older brothers.

I know I had no name until March of that year because in another letter I am referred to as "the baby." My brothers were to accompany me to New York City from our home at the far end of Singing Beach in Manchester-by-the-Sea, Massachusetts. That enormous brick house had been built for my grandmother, my father's mother. He had inherited it at the age of twenty-one when his mother was suddenly killed in an automobile crash.

In 1945, all four of us children moved into a duplex apartment on Park Avenue in Manhattan that my father had bought, sight unseen, for $40,000. He also invited his Great Aunt Nina, to live there, telling her that she could be "in charge of the staff."

When I was just two months old, my mother asked my grandmother to take me (alone for some reason) on that overnight train to Florida. My Uncle Arthur, Mummy's only sibling, told me this story several decades later. He said that both he and Mummy were "raging alcoholics." In fact, he once told me, "I don't know how in the world we made it to Florida alive, because your mother had only packed our suitcases with booze!"

I am glad I asked about this because I had never been told that my first outbreak of severe eczema occurred during that train ride. I doubt that my grandmother had ever taken care of me before, as I do know that there were always two nurses hired: one for the boys, referred to as "a tutor," and a nanny for the baby, me.

I was finally named for my mother, Alexandra, who was the fourth generation of Alexandras. My grandmother's grandfather had been a ship captain who sailed from Boston to Barcelona. He married Alexandra, according to family lore, after seeing her on the wharf and asking for an introduction.

In June of 1950, when I was still six, my stepmother married my father and chose to have me as her only attendant. The wedding was in the Harvard Chapel and the reception was in the faculty club. That is another vivid memory, partly, I suppose, because many photos were taken that day. I liked all the attention I got and remember standing up holding the bouquet and looking out at the congregation.

I became very close to my stepmother. She developed interests in child psychology and integrative medicine, and, after I had had all four of my children, she invited me to the Rockefeller home for a board meeting of the Institute for the Advancement of Health. The woman who funded that organization was Eileen Growald, who kindly allowed me to attend her board meeting. Eileen's father was David Rockefeller. I met many of the luminaries of integrated medicine from that era: Michael Lerner, Rachel Naomi Remen, Norman Cousins, Joan Borysenko, Dean Ornish, and Ken Pelletier, to brag about a few. I was fascinated by the mind, body, and spirit connections and how these threads were braided through my life.

During the summer when I was ten, I met Dr. Richard Hoffman, who was then considered the best dermatologist in all of Boston, which really meant the best in the world. Mummy had made an appointment for me at the Beth Israel Hospital the day after I arrived that summer after fifth grade.

Spending time with Dr. Hoffman became a highlight. Even our first meeting is memorable because he asked my mother to stay in the waiting room. He took me into a place where I think we were sitting side by side on a stretcher. What I know happened was that he took my hand and stroked it as he asked me questions. I had been to many dermatologists during this first decade of my eczema-focused life, but it was the first time I felt listened to and cared about.

Dr. Hoffman, after listening for who knows how long, said, "You know, Alexandra… I think this eczema has a lot to do with those brothers of yours." I knew he was right. I guess I told him about their incessant teasing and how they were always fighting. Then he asked, "How would you feel about coming into the hospital tomorrow? I want to get this to not bother you so much."

That month in the Beth Israel Hospital was the happiest month of my childhood. I got constant attention from the nurses, and Dr. Hoffman's visits were a steady delight. My skin did improve after a few weeks of tar treatments. The twice-daily application of tar lotion was very painful because it had an alcohol base and I had open sores all over my entire body. But the soothing tar cream afterward felt wonderful. Tar oil was applied to my scalp just at night, but soon it felt good, and I was no longer pulling out my hair. The regiment continued over the following year.

❋ ❦ ❋ ❦ ❋

*Listening to another's story somehow gives
us the strength of example to carry on, as
well as showing us aspects of ourselves we
can't easily see. For listening to the stories
of others ... is a kind of water that breaks the
fever of our isolation.*

—Mark Nepo

In 1981, I attended a well-run workshop by Joan Borysenko in Brookline, Massachusetts. I was eager to learn to meditate more regularly, so off I drove at night for the class that began at 8:00 p.m. I had to drive over forty minutes to get there and park in what I thought was a scary garage. Both ideas were stressful, but I was determined.

When I walked into the large room, I immediately saw that all the attendees were women. One was wearing a large straw hat, and I just knew I would be paired off with her. I mean, who wears a hat at night?

The workshop was full of strangers, except for Joan. She asked us to pair off, and, indeed, my intuition was correct—this weird straw-hatted lady was my partner for the workshop. When she saw my nametag, she lit up. "Are you related to Alexandra?" she asked.

I was astonished and simply responded, "Yes, that is my mother. How do you know her?"

"Oh, well, my father has had a crush on your mother for so many decades now," she said with a blush.

"And who is your father?" I asked incredulously.

"My dad is the pharmacist at the drug store in Manchester, Massachusetts," she answered.

I had talked with my oldest brother just the day before about our mother and the fact that she had so many medications all prescribed under different names. Mummy had now been married to her third husband for six years. At that particular time, she was in the Phillips House of Mass General Hospital with a vague diagnosis of "a swallowing problem."

I told my brother that through her hospitalization I was able to examine her medications, and I was bewildered as to the dates on the bottles. They had all been prescribed over the most recent couple of years, but the names she had used were from when she was married to our father.

The next time I visited Mummy was the day she was released. I was able to have a brief conversation with a nice older nurse who told me that in all her years of working at Phillips House she had never seen a worse case of delirium tremens, or alcohol withdrawal syndrome.

Another time, I visited Mummy in Manchester, along with her third husband, Bert. Bert was in the little room at the bottom of the stairs and had a fire going. He offered me a drink and had just sat down when Mummy came downstairs and sat next to me on the sofa.

"Mummy, can I get you anything?" I asked.

"I'd love a glass of milk," she replied.

I stood to go to the kitchen when Bert stopped me gently. "Don't fill it. Just pour half a glass."

When I returned and started to hand it to Mummy, Bert intercepted it. He gently took it, turned to the bar next to him, and quietly poured in half a glass of Jack Daniels bourbon. I said nothing but watched as he handed her the glass, now full, and said, "There you go, my dear."

To my astonishment, Mummy drank it down all at once! I was thunderstruck and did not say a word. Later, I told my brother about it, but we never did anything.

A month later, I visited Mummy again because she was not doing well. I knew that talking to her about important things would serve both of us well, so I told her that I knew we had loved each other as best we could and that I knew she loved me. I wanted her to know I would be fine after she left and assured her that she should feel free to die now. Telling her that my three older brothers also loved her, I explained that all of us were beginning to understand that everyone does the best they can in any given moment.

I was able to have a peaceful last visit with Mummy. She died three days later. That time when I had lain next to her in her bed had been very leisurely and comfortable, which was rather a miracle because there were not many times when we were together that we both felt relaxed, much less comfortable. I felt good about the fact that I was able to spend that time with her.

*　❀　*　❀　*

As a child I was brave, and because I needed attention so badly I would do anything to please my three older brothers. One day in Manchester, when I was three years old, I remember being dared to eat five large black ants.

The four of us were just outside the front door of "Stoneleigh," the house we had come to for our summer with our mother. We all crouched down to look at these enormous ants. My three older brothers told me that I had to eat five of them. I squished one, put it in my mouth, started to chew it, picked up another, did the same, and kept chewing till all five were gone. They all yelled their enthusiastic responses in astonishment. I was so pleased because I had not even tasted those ants but made my brothers proud.

*　❀　*　❀　*

Looking back on my childhood, I can see I had an unnourishing upbringing. I always felt a gnawing dissatisfaction, along with a yearning for comfortable relationships. I found those only in my non-family female friendships.

My mother saw us only in the summer, from mid-June to the end of August. My father sent us up to visit her with a female "sitter," who Mummy called "the spy." I suppose my father was concerned about Mummy's drinking. She had, after all, been in three different places "to be dried out," we were told. Astonishingly, my three older brothers and I were unaware of Mummy being an alcoholic.

At the end of May, in preparation for our arrival, Mummy would have whoever was cooking for her prepare sandwiches for me and my brothers for the entire summer and store them in one of the three large deep freezers (the other two freezers held potato chips and cigarettes, respectively). They were chicken salad sandwiches, made from canned chicken and Cain's Mayonnaise. Every morning after breakfast, I'd grab a frozen sandwich from the deep freeze, and put it in my bicycle basket to thaw during my "outing class" at the Essex County Club. At lunchtime, I would wash it down with a ten-cent Coke from the vending machine near the tennis courts.

For dinner, Mummy always had someone else prepare our meals. I particularly remember Mrs. Gates, who would come in the afternoon and get dinner ready for Mummy to put in the oven. She always left a note for Mummy (who was frequently sunbathing at the beach club), telling her what temperature to set the oven, how long to cook the meat, and how long to heat up the vegetables.

The worst dinner I can remember was the purple, gelatinous lamb. She obviously didn't read or follow Mrs. Gates' directions properly because it was raw. Why my stepfather did not ask Mummy to put that meat back in the oven, I don't know. It was likely that he already had a sufficient amount of Do Good bourbon to make him either not notice or not care. He would carve all the meat at the sideboard and then create a salad course. He seemed to enjoy dragging out the ritual of making the salad dressing, which he did at the table in the large wooden spoon of the salad servers. He would stir a little dried mustard with the olive oil and lots of salt and pepper. I have never liked salad.

We all managed to say nothing about the food, as my mother frequently left the table to have "a quiet little puke" in the downstairs bathroom. When we had corn on the cob, fresh from my stepfather's garden, my brothers and I would compete over who could devour the most ears of corn. I won several times and loved the role of winner, but most of the time I left the dinner table hungry.

Back in NYC, where he had custody of all of us the rest of the year, my father hired Anna Lundgren from Sweden, who cooked for my family for twenty-three years. I liked Anna a lot, and she prepared pretty good meals for us. But I always wanted more meat.

When my father would carve the roast on a sideboard, he would ask me to pass each plate to everyone else. When I finally got my plate, it had only a tiny portion. He insisted that I wait until everyone else had their second helpings before allowing me more meat. Also, because my eczema was sufficiently bad, I had been put on a restrictive diet as early as age three. I was not allowed eggs, wheat, or citrus fruits, among so much more. I remember trying to eat food off others' plates just to taste the eggs. To this day, when I pick up a delicious, cooked chicken, I am apt to eat most of it all by myself before it gets cold. My father hated to waste food, and I feel the same way. He was devoted to each of his eight children, and we all loved him.

I did not much enjoy the years of cooking for my husbands, nor did I like going out for dinner parties. Food has been an issue forever, and now I am used to being both gluten- and dairy-free. I am so euphoric over having no more eczema that I still eat to be fed more than to enjoy the meal.

I have disliked cooking for many years and now, thank God, have Monica to prepare my food. She dislikes cooking as much as I do, but we laugh about it and manage to get ourselves fed. As my daughter pointed out, I am always glad to have a meal over with!

❊ ❦ ❊ ❦ ❊

I am now seventy-eight years old, and I am still studying how having severe eczema has affected me. Two sons and one daughter have inherited my condition, and for the past decade I have focused on my unsolved mystery of how to get over it. Now I am living with barely a trace, and it has improved the most during this pandemic. Winifred Marion, a Chinese medical Qigong practitioner, tells me I can look at both the steroid creams and the inner work (the energy work I do with moving meridians with The Dragon's Way) as solutions to keep from further suffering.

I am now convinced the major problem for my eczema is unexpressed emotions. I accept that I have inherited the tendency toward this skin condition, as both of my parents had it and all three of my older brothers also suffered from psoriasis and eczema, though a great deal less severely than I have. Five years ago, I went off eating gluten and dairy. I realize that it may not be for everyone, but for me that has done a lot to cure my skin. I will continue to keep to my restricted diet and pray that expressing my emotions will help keep my skin feeling good and healthy. Now I am able to be aware of my anger and sadness. At last, I can feel them in my body. I now want to exercise and strive for four days a week.

I trust life now. I look at nature. I choose to believe there is an afterlife. I ask for help from my Guides or Angels, and I believe they do provide it! My gratitude to my companion Monica is so deep that I attribute most of how I now feel to living with her unconditional acceptance and love for me. She never criticizes me or tells me how I ought to be. This is the motherly love that I did not get, and how extraordinary to discover that it is never too late!

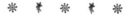

If I gave my eczema a voice, I sense it may say the following:

> Hello, Alexandra, I am glad to be asked to put in my take on this lifelong effort to help you. I am a part of you that you are beginning to listen to. I know you like the image of a Healing Circle, so here is what I would like you to do.
>
> Imagine that you are the host of your Healing Circle out there in your backyard. You have around you the members of your former board of trustees. You no longer call yourself Chairman of the Board but Host of the Circle, which will help you continue to heal.

I am one of the voices you need to listen to very carefully. I have gotten a great deal of attention over the decades, but now is the perfect time for you to honestly hear what I am telling you.

Put very simply, I represent unexpressed emotions. You were not able to act out all the feelings of sadness and loss you experienced as an infant and toddler. I came into your life, as you know, when you were a small baby. Every doctor you were taken to wanted me to vanish. But I am here to help you learn how to feel and express in healthy ways the feelings that got cut off when you were a child. It is not too late, dear Alexandra, for you to learn to feel the feelings.

I am so happy to know you are now going to see Winifred for her Chinese medical approach. She will continue to give you treatments and include Qigong as part of your practice. The exercises will help you develop more feeling in your body. They will also release some of the residue of the "red skin syndrome" that accumulated from your overuse of cortisone. You have been tolerant about the recurrence of a red splotchy face, and I am glad because you will need to go through more of this slow releasing of what was stored.

When you see the phenomenal closeness Monica has with her family, you have such a big question about why you have the relationship with your family that you do. I know this because you speak of it often, and I think you will see that part of it is that in her culture, family is number one in importance. In the culture you were born into, family is considered important, but being popular is also highly valued.

As I think of you as a ten-year-old at the Spence School and remember how well-liked you were, I wonder if that was an area you found easy to excel in. You knew you could not compete in the academic arena, but you found making friends very easy. My hope is that now that you have become more discerning in your friendships, you will no longer feel you need to have what one of your therapists called "100 percent friends."

You are really doing well, and I am so pleased to notice the steps you have taken to heal yourself. Your ability to listen to your intuition has improved this past decade, and you sought out long-distance healing for yourself. Then you went to The Biomed Center up in Providence, which was remarkably effective, only you did not anticipate months of "red rash syndrome" (nor did they). But you kept at it and now realize the importance of emoting!

I know Winifred has encouraged you to watch sad movies to get you to cry. You still find it hard to do the deep sobbing that I want to see. But I am patient, and I believe you are really on the path to heal more and more. You are becoming increasingly aware of who you are and what that means for your choices. I will always be a part of you, reminding you to slow down and assisting you in breaking the old habit, for example, of rushing all day long.

It is such a delight to notice how much you are appreciating my *not* bothering you. Although the splotchy face reminds you of me, you are well aware that it is not itchy. I know you are self-conscious about not looking your absolute best, but I promise you, if you just relax, you will realize you emit an energy that is unique and contains a lot of serenity.

Your presence is enough, Alexandra. I love being your protector. I see so much improvement, so just know that I will continue to watch over you and congratulate you. You are now doing less multitasking and way less rushing around everywhere. I see you actually feeling your body being relaxed, noticing it, and being grateful. So please keep up your efforts. I am here and will let you know when you need to be reminded of my benevolent presence.

※ ❋ ※ ❋ ※

Today I am feeling hopeful. On the physical level, I have an outbreak of eczema on my face, neck, scalp, and ears, but it is not terrible. It is red now, as I just put on an olive-oil-based pure salve that my daughter-in-law made as part of home schooling her daughters, aged 7 and 8. It turns out to be the one cream that soothes and does not create itching. I will put on another cream after my shower, and that one is called EUCRISA®. I have a new dermatologist who gives me samples of this cream because my insurance will not cover the nearly $800 per small tube. (He prescribed an alternative one but the pharmacist at CVS told me it would cost $2000!) This tiny tube of what looks like Vaseline actually does calm the redness. I slather it on after my shower and then it stings like bloody hell, but I reapply it several more times during the day.

This shows that I still rely on Western medicine for help and that I have an impressive number of supplements that I take daily. When I consulted with a nutritionist named Josh Boughton, he mentioned a powder called "GI Globulin Select™" that I now put a small scoop of in my morning smoothie, and it has made my digestion phenomenally better.

The day before yesterday, I went in for my first visit to Master Nan Lu's office in Manhattan, and there I received a treatment from his acupuncturist, Tatiana. She was a caring practitioner who took my pulse and said I have very good energy, which I am aware of feeling. She was able to discern how my liver and other organs are faring and prescribed some helpful herbs that I take morning and night. I need not get into the particulars, because the main point is that I have chosen to believe that my daily Qigong practice is helping me.

Tatiana also told me to stay away from chicken for a while and instead eat a lot of fish (but not shrimp) and mung beans, which I will order. Naturally, fruits and vegetables are encouraged, and having Monica here to help me with cooking I will do my best. The good news from Tatiana was that I should never become a vegetarian because I need the nutrients of red meat. The two times I tried to do just veggies I became anemic. My body needs that source of protein, and learning this was a relief because I had been feeling slightly guilty about my reluctance to avoid red meat.

I am now aware of being able to say "no" to things I am not interested in doing, and I can feel my body in a relaxed state for far more of the day. I definitely feel more confident, and this is enabling me to speak more directly and be less apt to try and figure out why someone is behaving differently toward me. In the past I would take that someone aside and see if I could repair a possible hurt that I might have inflicted. Now I just accept that that person is dealing as best they can with their new boundaries. I accept the situation and no longer need everyone I know to like me. I am conscious of changing how I interact with friends and allowing how I feel in the moment to dictate my behavior, and I like the freedom that this gives me.

Yes, I am feeling better both physically and emotionally. After some time away from the practice, I decided to recommit to Qigong when my skin started acting up. The redness was so bad one day that I began doubting whether my decision to follow Master Lu's practice was really doing anything. But I decided to watch a sad movie when Winifred said I need to cry more and get out the tears from my past that I never shed. After crying while watching the movie that afternoon, I suddenly felt nauseous and ran to the bathroom where I violently vomited and had explosive diarrhea. When I looked in the mirror after that episode, I saw that my skin was no longer inflamed. This got my attention, so I decided to recommit to Master Lu's Chinese medical Qigong! This is also why I wanted to receive acupuncture, and Tatiana is continuing to address the inflammation that shows on my skin.

I believe we can heal ourselves more than I previously understood. In time, I am hopeful that the rash will actually disappear, and I will attribute the success to following this regimen. I feel my aliveness as never before, my vitality is way up, and now I truly love my life.

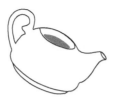

CHAPTER 3

Longing to Be Liked

I began to see that each person's story,
no matter how different than my own,
would suddenly be about a part of me that
I had never given voice to.

—Mark Nepo

There was a lot of talk about stopping at two children, as was socially acceptable, but my husband and I really wanted a third. So, we did not talk about it a lot, and I was slightly embarrassed at some NYC gatherings where I knew I was looked at as a pregnant woman with a bit of condemnation. But I had a mercifully easy pregnancy, and when the day of May 14, 1973, arrived, I was very happy.

We did not know whether this baby was going to be a boy or a girl, but, either way, it would have an older brother and sister, each about two years apart. I spent several hours in labor in the Boston Hospital for Women. The two previous births had been at Lenox Hill Hospital in NYC, and I had been completely unconscious for the first child's birth and had the second naturally. This time my doctor persuaded me to have an epidural. The obstetrician told me his wife had had one and that he was a big fan, so I agreed to be given this injection.

What I had not predicted was being left alone in the room after the nurse put the huge epidural needle in my back. My body became increasingly colder, and I could not seem to find a way to call the nurse. When she finally came in I was relieved, but when she took my blood pressure she said, "Oh no! This is terrible. You are *way* too low," and shouted for a nurse to come in.

I became terrified because I was freezing cold and no one was speaking to me. I was rushed up to the delivery room and, weirdly, as soon as I was given blankets, all the excitement was gone. My husband was not allowed in to watch the birth, just as he had not been allowed in for the first two deliveries. I felt completely abandoned and alone, even though the doctor was present. There was no camaraderie like there had been with my natural childbirth, which had been exciting because I was awake and could participate. With this birth I was also awake, but I remember thinking it was sort of like going for a pedicure because it felt like I was receiving a service more than having a baby. There was no one encouraging or supporting me.

When I was told that I had a baby girl, I was thrilled. But the doctor did not give her to me to hold because he said she was a little "floppy" and that they were going to keep her on watch for a bit. I did not know what to think. I was not sure what this meant but asked if it was due to the kind of anesthesia I had been given. I was told that it might be. They were not sure yet.

I was taken to the recovery room and from there up to my room. My husband left at that point and said he would be busy as he had a meeting he needed to attend, so once again, I felt very alone. It was strange to feel so isolated during such a momentous event.

At 9:00 p.m. the obstetrician appeared at my door to tell me that my little girl had jaundice. He said they were moving her into the special care nursery and would keep a close eye on her. He repeated that she was very lethargic and not responding as rapidly as they expected. I was frightened and wanted to call my husband, but having been asked to not call him, I decided I needed to be alone with my worry. Later, I discovered that many babies were affected from their mothers being given an epidural.

I had trouble sleeping that night and did not ask a lot of questions. All I remember is praying for this little baby. While I was in labor, her father and I had been discussing what to name her. We had an easy time with a boy's name but debated a lot about a female name. Finally, we selected the name Rachel.

My mother-in-law had been a Shaw, and it was her mother that we named Rachel after. That ancestor had been politically active even in her eighties and apparently had a wonderful husband who encouraged her to speak out at Quaker meetings in Philadelphia. Her family was proud of her leading the First Continental Congress with Susan B. Anthony. What impressed me the most, however, was that this ancestor of my baby girl was also one of the white women who helped make the Underground Railroad work. I had spent my youth going to a family plantation in South Carolina, so I saw firsthand the poverty of the Black families who worked for our family.

I hoped my daughter would be proud of her ancestor, and that her influence would positively impact her character. It is funny to look back now on how little I knew. Now I realize how little we understand about the influence a name can have on a child. I think we were lucky, and our Rachel has carried her name with pride, but just how good or bad it was for her, I have no idea.

The morning after Rachel's birth, I was able to breastfeed her, and when I saw her sweet little face, albeit a bit yellow, I was so relieved to feel love for her as instantaneously as I had for her siblings.

The pediatrician later came in and told me his wife had had the same "floppy baby" after being given an epidural. He was convinced that the blocker did not have a negative impact on the baby; at least he assured me that his daughter was now fine and that he expected Rachel would be too.

❈　❀　❈　❀　❈

Each year, starting at age three, my three older brothers and I were sent up from NYC to the North Shore of Massachusetts. Our mother lived there with her husband, whom she married just before I turned three in June of 1946. We were not invited to her wedding.

The driveway where they lived was steep, and their car would go all the way to the top where there was a circular driveway with huge rhododendrons in the center. My father would drop us off there with all our luggage. I hated saying goodbye to him, and he never went up to the door with us. My oldest brother, John, was the one who would run up to ring the bell and call Mummy. She would come out, but we all knew the only one she was really delighted to see was her firstborn.

I no longer have a sense of what happened which summer, but the images of particular events are still vivid and make me glad to remember them. The first memory is all four of us deciding to throw apples through each of the many windows in the three-car garage, which was a fair distance from the big gray house that overlooked the ocean. Mummy and our step-father were off visiting someone that afternoon, leaving us four children in this huge house with its three-car garage—all on our own. Funnily enough, it is one of my happiest childhood memories. We hurled apples with real glee and broke every last pane in each window in that garage structure. It was the only time I can recall a sense of connection between all four of us, and we got away with it.

Another time my brother Beek and I pulled up all the vegetables from my stepfather's extensive garden. He had a very kind gardener named Cooney, and I am surprised that we punished him when our aim was to infuriate our stepfather. I remember how satisfied we all were that we took something with so much structure and order and messed it up. Later, my stepfather yelled at us, sent us upstairs to our separate rooms, and told us we would have no dinner that night. But Mummy felt sorry for us, and I remember her bringing me food on a tray. I presume she did the same for Beek.

Years later, Beek and I were talking late into the night and heard Mummy leaving her room, as she was very heavy-footed. We switched off the light and watched as she entered a guest room near where we were standing. There was a full moon over the ocean, and we could see Mummy unlock the bureau drawer and remove a flask. She then tipped it up so she could drink it down, and we could actually hear the gulps! We were transfixed by this. It was the first time our eyes were opened to her drinking, and we were fifteen and eighteen years old! We had been told that Mummy had a "drinking problem" and that she had gone to several hospitals (psychiatric ones, we later discovered) "to be dried out," but none of us realized that her problem had persisted.

Beek and I stayed up discussing what we should do, and this led to a permanent rift between Beek and Mummy. The next morning Mummy was in bed and very contrite. Having discussed how to handle what we had seen, Beek and I designated Beek as the spokesperson, who announced that she should go to Alcoholics Anonymous and that our stepfather should take her. But there was a lot of resistance, and Beek told them both that he was going to leave if they refused to follow this counsel. I, loving my brother Beek a great deal, said I would leave with him. I cannot remember where I went, but I did stay away for a few weeks. I felt sorry for Mummy, but Beek never returned.

Every time I saw my mother, she asked me how Beek was. We did not talk often on the phone, but, when we did, she would ask if Beek was okay. She lived until 1981, but Beek stayed away. When he died about five years ago, we were no longer close.

John, my oldest big brother, was literally referred to as "The Golden." Mummy did not seem to find anything wrong with labeling us. Her second born was Michael, and he was called "Lead."

Due to his brain damage, Michael was not able to graduate from Solebury School, the boarding school he was sent to for his high school years. He was a most unhappy person and occasionally got furious with his younger siblings, namely Beek and me. I especially remember that day he threw me down the stairs in our Park Avenue apartment in NYC and how no one scolded him or comforted me for that incident.

Beek was called "Silver" and I was called "Bronze." The first psychiatrist I saw as an adult asked if he could "borrow" the letters that Mummy sent me. She addressed her letters "Dear Bronze," not "Dear Daughter." I gave them to him because he told me he was going to present them at a psychiatric conference. Unfortunately, that psychiatrist suffered from a sleeping disorder. He not only nodded off during our sessions but never remembered to return my letters.

I can see now that Mummy was probably drinking when she repeatedly told me how she had only wanted one child, and that was John. She said she just did not want me and never had.

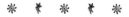

I wish to examine the habits that no longer serve me and the ones I wish to learn from. I think I understand from watching interviews with Gabor Maté that the drive to be close to someone is the biggest need for humans. Second to that is authenticity. He explains that this is what gets cut off when an infant attempts to attach to an overly stressed mother. When this happened to me, I tried to get my attention externally. The good news is I survived, but the bad news is that I became addicted to being liked. I was trying to get what I needed from others because I did not have the capacity to get it from within due to physical brain functions that could not happen when I was an infant. This information, in effect, takes me off the hook. I suppressed my own needs because I was not loved for who I was. Suppressing my needs also suppressed my immune system. I was always looking for love from the outside because I did not have it for myself on the inside. This means I lost my connection to my essence.

In his book *Seat of the Soul*, Michael Singer says that he believes our essence is our Soul, and that is what makes sense to me now. I am glad I am doing massage plus the energy treatments from Winifred because I now have the opportunity to discover whether I can gain the ability to feel deeply. It has only recently occurred to me that I am lacking this ability. I have also lost the "playfulness" ability.

I have also learned more about myself from *The Drama of the Gifted Child* by Alice Miller. I know I was, and still am, a sensitive Soul, so perhaps I can learn to listen to my Soul? I no longer resist the idea of my being gifted, and though I feel shy about saying I am creative, my desire to understand myself through Maté's lens is very strong. Even now, I am sitting here in my reading room listening to opera music while watching my neighbor paint her front porch steps and am wildly impressed by her doing so much each day. She is so skilled in many ways that help her maintain her house. I have totally different skills, but we share so much, such as our longtime desire to be well-liked and our ability to be so. When I think about authenticity, I think about what my skills and interests are and accept them without comparing them to others or judging them as wrong.

Looking at the transformative work I have chosen also shows me who I am authentically. Two chaplaincy training groups nineteen years apart and three years of hospice work show me I definitely have been eager to grow and change for the better. I did several Buddhist retreats and a few Christian ones as well. Mostly I wanted to help myself feel better and help others. I loved the opportunities to listen to people who wanted to talk about serious issues, often during the darkest times of their lives. My interest in social work also aligns with this. Winifred and I are hoping to take hospice training to become "end of life doulas" someday.

✽ ❉ ✽ ❉ ✽

I was at loose ends through all of my adolescence, so it is not surprising that I married at twenty-three and knew nothing. I chose to go to a boarding school because my three older brothers had all gone, and I guess I thought it was what one did. I was completely unaware of how my terrible academic record would hinder my choices. But honestly, I did not really know I was making choices about anything.

It is so odd to compare myself to two of my granddaughters who have been staying with me for nearly two weeks now. But they seem so confident and clear about what to do with their time. They both have Zoom requirements, exams, and classes, and they manage their food intake so effortlessly. I am in awe of their ability to stay connected to themselves; they seem to know who they are. I had no clue at their age.

One way to understand how "at loose ends" I was throughout my adolescent years is to recognize my need to be with friends all the time. I had no concept of a "me" that I could listen to and was simply buoyed by my friends. I had no idea why I was a showoff, for example, but one day an English teacher, Miss Baker, pulled me out of a gathering at the library after a talk by a man from the United Nations. All I can remember was wanting to get a laugh, so I blurted out something inappropriate, and Miss Baker told me to leave. We went into her classroom nearby and she was really angry. I had never seen her like this, and she startled me by saying, "What gets into you, Alexandra?"

I immediately felt shame, but it was a moment I will always be grateful for because I had never asked myself that question. Suddenly I saw that I desperately wanted and needed attention. I don't know if we talked; I only know that I knew she cared about me.

The lack of guidance from my parents has made me want to help people, teenagers in particular, sort out their lives. Funnily enough, my grandchildren don't seem to need it, but I benefit from their honesty. When I asked my nineteen-year-old granddaughter what it was like for her when I suggest books for her to read, she told me she really does not want to read anything but the books she chooses. What was so lovely for me was that she heard my frustration. I was hoping for a connection, and this conversation led to one. Just realizing that I want to have that connection helps me recognize that my adolescence lacked this. No wonder I felt "at loose ends."

My three years at Chatham Hall, the high school in southern Virginia, was a time of very little introspection. The one incident with Miss Baker was a highlight, and the other was at graduation. I was sitting on the stage way over to the left, looking out at the parents and faculty in the audience. The headmaster, an Episcopal minister, was giving the introduction before announcing the recipients of the three top honors in the school.

The first one was the head of the student council, a group in which I had not made even one of the ten possible spots. Then there was the Madonna award, a surprise announcement in chapel. The award recipient sat with a blue shawl over her shoulders and was holding a doll. To this day I don't know what the award was really about.

That June, something else extraordinary happened at graduation. The headmaster began describing how a girl had made the spirit of the school better and that this was the reason she was chosen to receive the honor. When he mentioned that she had made a wonderful Santa Claus, I gasped because I was the only one who had done that. It had never occurred to me that I could be given an honor, especially not a highly coveted one like the Rector's Medal, but here I was, about to get up and receive it!

I had not excelled in any sport or in any class, yet I was being given this huge congratulations. I was aware of my father and stepmother in the audience and knew they must have been as flabbergasted as my classmates were. This significant and positive jolt was very much the start of my rocky road to self-knowledge. I was so happy to discover that my older brother had received the equivalent at his boarding school, St. Mark's. Clearly we are extraordinarily alike in many, many ways. In fact, he and I have become close over the past few decades, and I am about to fly to Charleston to visit him and his dear wife. We will all attend the ceremony at the College of Charleston where he will be given an honorary degree in philanthropy.

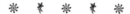

While sitting on two cushions in my dining room, I am looking at a large candle in the center of a circular table. I can see a smaller circular table outside with two matching wrought-iron chairs and my neighbor Mary putting things into her trunk. Happily, she and I have already had our walk this morning. Having a neighbor whom I like and can drop in on is a little slice of heaven during this pandemic.

This prompts me to write about Monica again, who, at this moment, is in the kitchen making us chicken soup. We hardly ever eat the same food, but we shop together and always buy two fully cooked chickens at Hannaford each week. Monica prefers fish and Caribbean food, so she gets plantains and cooks a separate meal for herself. We eat together at the butcher block island in the kitchen.

Yesterday, two friends dropped in on Monica and me. To my delight, we all sat in my reading room, which has a sectional sofa with an ottoman. We made ourselves comfy, putting our feet up on the ottoman, and had such a pleasant and interesting chat for nearly an hour. I realized then that Monica had not joined us in this room before. She is recognizing that we want her to be with us, and I can tell she is liking our interactions a lot.

I am the first "job" Monica has had taking care of someone who is not sick. She cooks, cleans, and does all kinds of things. Today she hemmed a pair of pants that needed it. We have become good friends, although I do recognize that she is being paid to look after me. If my other friends are over, she usually discreetly goes upstairs or into another room, but with these two good friends she is comfortable being with us.

What is so interesting is how our friendship has changed both of us. I truly know that I am more grounded, in part because of Monica. I think it may be her strong faith in God. When anyone meets her, the depth of her kindness shows up immediately. She is at peace. She listens to prayers for a long time each morning before she comes down to make her coffee in the small drip coffee maker. There is a calmness about Monica. Her trust in good overcoming evil is something I am sure affects me. She is sharing her faith with me, and I feel less insecure and more able to relax than I used to.

After I moved here eight years ago, my neighbor asked if I would like to come to a meditation group that she had been going to every Thursday at 5:30 p.m. for five years. I said I would give it a try and found I liked the group and the way the guided meditation was conducted. When Monica was asked if she would join this meditation group, sixteen months ago now, she agreed to give it a try. She already knew a few of the ladies, so it was easier than it might have been otherwise. We have gone regularly ever since, but now, with COVID-19, the group has temporarily stopped meeting.

Monica is incredibly devoted to her family. Every night she calls her mother and siblings in St. Lucia and usually talks with them for at least an hour. In fact, just before Thanksgiving she will be leaving to visit them for about six weeks and will quarantine down there in order to be able to spend Christmas with her family.

Last weekend I drove Monica to visit one of her closest friends, a woman named Esther who is from her same poor neighborhood in St. Lucia. I had communicated with Esther because she had given me two books after Monica visited her in Goshen, but I had not met her until last Sunday. I was fascinated to find how easily we could talk, the three of us. Monica told me that their mothers had been very good friends, and Esther has kept in close touch with Monica ever since Monica came to the US in 1990.

Esther went to college and then medical school to become an allergist. She married a Jewish professor when she was thirty-eight. When I interviewed Monica for this job, she explained that she was looking after Esther's husband until he died. After his death, Esther moved to a smaller place, and this is where we drove last weekend.

Somehow the fact that my privileged white background has not prevented me from feeling comfortable with two women of similar early childhoods but different education levels makes me hopeful. It was clear to Monica that Esther and I liked one another, and I am so deeply grateful for this new person in my life. The first book Esther gave me was *The Color of Water* by James McBride. This book about the upbringing of a poor Black boy in NYC was such a fascinating one. The author's mother provided for her twelve children, all of whom went to college and earned graduate degrees. The book I brought to Esther was *Caste* by Isabel Wilkerson. What I treasure is that the three of us are educating each other despite the contrast of our very different backgrounds.

❋ ❋ ❋ ❋ ❋

Yesterday I had a conversation with one of my sons for over an hour. One of the topics was my realization that treating my two boys differently than my two girls may be one reason I have such a difficult relationship with my daughters. This was, of course, an unconscious process. But with all the awareness of racial bias in our culture, I am beginning to realize that I probably had a bias as well: albeit unintentionally, I showed more respect for maleness.

My son told me that he had just that week pointed out to his mother-in-law that she was asking the three men at dinner what they thought about an issue. He stopped her to point out that she had not asked her daughter (his wife), who was sitting right there, her opinion on the matter. My son told me that neither his mother-in-law nor I think we are very smart, but the truth is we are both highly intelligent. Then he explained his view of intelligence. He said that intelligence in general, the type equivalent to being adept at crossword puzzles, is fine but that emotional intelligence, the type his mother-in-law and I possess, is far more important.

Now, in April of 2022, I am recognizing the impact of my childhood longings on my children. My desire to be seen and understood led me to unconsciously request recognition from my children. I was needing connection and did not realize that this put a wedge into my relationships, especially with my daughters. Sometimes they felt they were not enough, and I was oblivious to my role in those feelings. As Brené Brown states, "We need to dispel the myth that empathy is 'walking in someone else's shoes.' Rather than walking in your shoes, I need to learn how to listen to the story you tell about what it's like in your shoes and believe you even when it doesn't match my experiences."[2]

* * * * *

"What absorbs you so completely that you know it is central to your own healing?"

This question startles me because I have been ruminating on why I was so fascinated by watching the Summit on Collective Trauma on the internet. I am curious when something grabs my attention so powerfully whether it is leading me to more healing. And I think it is.

The very first speaker at the summit captivated me. Her name is Jacqueline Novogratz, and her newest book is titled *Manifesto for a Moral Revolution: Practices to Build a Better World*. She is the founder and CEO of Acumen, a company she started nineteen years ago. Through Acumen, entrepreneurs and investors worldwide have built a community that brings clean water, sanitation, energy, healthcare, and education to hundreds of millions of low-income people. *Forbes* magazine named Jacqueline Novogratz one of the world's 100 greatest living minds.[3]

---

2. Brené Brown, *Atlas of The Heart: Mapping Meaningful Connection and the Language of Human Experience* (New York: Random House, 2021), 123.

3. Acumen, "*Forbes* Names Jacqueline Novogratz as one of 100 Greatest Living Business Minds," September 19, 2017, https://acumen.org/blog/

Why is this such a pull on my attention? I think my own healing will enhance my ability to connect people in mutually beneficial ways. One of my major gifts is my ability to connect people. I am fortunate in knowing many people who are passionate about being a part of positive change, and many also have enormous resources.

Also, I have always noticed the discrepancy of wealth. I grew up spending vacations at a plantation in South Carolina where I felt very affected by the poverty of the Black workers who waited on us. As a child I saw their homes and was aware of the disparity between us. And, I have always been impressed when I read that it takes a collective will to eliminate poverty.

❋ ❦ ❋ ❦ ❋

I am wondering how the rest of the world is coping with this time of isolation. I am blessed in myriad ways and feel so bewildered by the news. My personal good fortune has me living peacefully in Rhinebeck, NY, with plenty of friends and neighbors able to visit. What is clear to me is how little I know or understand about this life. I am writing today about my own experience with family members and friends who have struggled with

forbes-names-jacqueline-novogratz-as-one-of-100-greatest-living-business-minds/.

mental illness. For ease of reading, and to protect their privacy, I have changed their names and how they are connected to me.

A friend named Julie developed an eating disorder when she was attending St. Timothy's School in Maryland. This led to some psychiatric issues that I was never told about. She was a model at one point and an excellent horseback rider. She never married and seemed very reclusive. What sticks in my memory is that her mother was a Christian Scientist and her father an alcoholic. This made an impression on me because this same combination of an alcoholic husband and Christian Scientist wife showed up another time in my life. And the similarities did not end there. In both cases, the combo emphasized denial in a big way.

Another couple also had a daughter, whose name is Charlene. I barely knew her even though my brothers and I spent our summers in the same town of Beverly Farms, MA, with our mother. Charlene lived with her parents, who lived next door to Charlene's grandmother, Gaga, whom we visited every day. We would occasionally see her and her family at the Singing Beach Club where we went often. She was five years younger than me, pretty, and smart.

Charlene went off to private school and developed an eating disorder, again something I knew nothing about. In those times, no one ever acknowledged disabilities or mental illness of any kind. Years later, we wound up living in the same town yet again. It was then that I reached out and got to know this sad, lonely woman. She lived in a house with fourteen dogs, and the Board of Health finally closed their home. She then went to another psychiatric hospital, as did her husband. They later divorced after having two daughters.

When she came home for Thanksgiving during her first year of college, Charlene told me she announced to her parents that she had found a therapist. Her parents (the alcoholic and the Christian Scientist) forbade her to return to therapy. In response, she went down to the police station and took off all her clothes to get the attention and help she needed. She told me this story with humor and added that she should have done some research because she was put into the worst facility in MA. She had about fifty more hospitalizations, and none were as bad as that first one. Her brother told me that she had been psychotic for seven years before she was placed in the assisted living facility she now calls home. We talk or text every weekend, and I have visited her several times.

I am riveted by the importance of bonding as well as genetics. I mention this because our family and close friends are certainly privileged and have been able to secure the best available treatments for mental and physical diseases, yet we are a rather unhealthy bunch. This topic leaves me with more questions than answers and is important to me in unlocking my own struggles with gut issues and eczema. I see how our bodies do keep score and how that shows up differently for different people. Maybe it is part of our journey to discover this for ourselves.

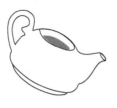

CHAPTER 4

Navigating Relationships

I would never compare my husbands to dogs. That is not at all what this is about. Rather, it is about how I navigated these relationships the way I navigate life: recklessly. The thread that pulls these stories together is my own beliefs and social norms, wrapped together with the fantasy of how I thought they should look.

Dogs are so smart. Even without words they have communicated so vividly to me. I have always seen them as something that could provide me company. I had an image of what dog ownership was going to look like, and it involved companionship and not so much training and discipline.

I bought my first dog in 1964. She was a Lhasa Apso, a breed known for being exotic, and was elegant and well-balanced. I named her Eva after my beloved nanny who was sent away when I was seven because my stepmother was jealous of our relationship.

I had not had a dog growing up, yet I always wanted one. By age twenty-one, I could finally buy myself a dog. I was going to San Francisco State College at the time, and it worked out so well because she, little Eva, loved children. I would leave her at the daycare center on the campus, and the teachers happily took charge of her running in the playground because it enchanted the children and made my puppy so happy.

One day, I took little Eva in for her check-up and distemper shot. Later at home, she had a seizure. When I brought her back to the vet, I was told she had to be put to sleep. So that was the dramatic and tragic end of my first dog's life.

For three months of every year, for three or four years before our divorce, my first husband was gone from 7:00 a.m. to 3:00 a.m. the following morning. I never questioned it, and those last few years I adapted to not having him around. It was not like he was with us much anyway. When he was home, he spent time in the basement doing carpentry or, that last year, building us a garage. He was absent both emotionally and phys-ically, and the children and I went on vacations without him, so I was used to him not being present.

We met in December of 1965 when he was about to start law school at Columbia University and I was taking courses in the general studies program there.

We dated for a few months and got married in September of 1966.

I knew little to nothing about marriage—or about being an adult, for that matter. When I moved into the apartment on East 63rd Street in Manhattan, I did not realize I would need a vacuum cleaner. When I had this young man over for dinner, I burned the quail that I had bought to impress him.

I had done very little reading, apart from true romance magazines, and paid almost no attention during all my years of schooling, despite attending a private boarding school following a private girls' school in the city. I adored musicals and thought that I would be able to "love, honor, and obey" whatever man I fell in love with. I was utterly ignorant about the impact that my inherited money would have upon any marriage, as it did with each of my three marriages.

This first husband and I had four children together, two years apart, and it was not until we were out celebrating our fifteenth anniversary that I asked him if he would rather be celebrating with someone else. He answered "Yes, I would. Would you?"

I told him, "No, but I feel very disconnected from you."

Three months later we went on a business trip to Acapulco. On the way into the hotel, I asked my husband if he wanted a divorce. He said yes, he did. I then asked to not join the group of his colleagues for dinner, but to eat in our room. We did, and it never occurred to me to fight to keep him. Nor did it occur to me that he had fallen in love with his secretary. Our children were six, eight, ten, and twelve at the time we divorced.

Despite the era, I was financially able to leave not only this marriage but the next two. Today I recognize my need to speak of my privilege. Part of why I stayed in the third marriage was because I felt more accepted when I could take the arm of a man. I feared I would be viewed with pity or disgust if I were alone.

I loved having my four children and taking care of them, and I focused on them and not on my husband. When he no longer wanted to be with me, I consciously made the decision to withdraw any energy that would feed his ego. It was not drastic, but it made an impact. We were divorced within months.

My second dog entered my life more than a decade later. I had just separated from my first husband who did not like dogs and refused to get one even though my children and I wanted one. Now that I was alone with the kids, we decided to get a family dog—a lab. I liked the idea of my children having a beloved dog, as I had adored my brother's dog, Tessie, whom we only saw on vacations in South Carolina. I named this puppy after a cousin I like named Annie.

Even my friends who loved labs wondered if we had gotten a lemon. Annie was impossible to train, and she chewed everything in sight. She destroyed my son

Michael's record player, and each morning there was a poop waiting for me in the kitchen. Once, while we were outside welcoming Michael home from a trip, Annie ate the cake we had made for him.

I became particularly desperate when Annie became so rambunctious in "puppy school" that I dropped out, but I really did not understand about training at all. I am also a "once over lightly" kind of person, and therefore struggled with the consistency required for good training.

I even hired a dog shrink to come for a home visit. His recommendation was clear: "You just put her bed in this small bathroom, put the leash on her, and shut this door. In the morning, you take her out. This will make her learn where she is meant to relieve herself."

That next morning, I was excited for no poop in the kitchen, but the foul smell from the bathroom hit me before I could open the door. Annie had bitten through her leash, vomited, pooped on her bed, and made a disgusting mess of that tiny bathroom! I had already paid the pet shrink and felt defeated.

Then one day, my dear friend Kathy who lives in Bermuda called. "I have a solution for you, Alexandra. I have the runt of our litter of Lhasa Apsos. I think Annie just needs a pal, and this little companion will make her happy."

Why I agreed to this, I cannot recall, but we named this puppy Theodora and called her Theo. She was as enchanting as Eva had been, and she lived even after all her vaccinations.

But the combination of the two dogs did not resolve things for me. The woman who cleaned for us in Lincoln, MA, came up with a truly welcome solution. "My brother adores dogs, and he can take her out hunting and give her plenty of exercise."

Annie was now fully grown and had been a constant nuisance for several years, so no one objected to this solution. In fact, I don't recall any resistance to Annie going to her new "forever home." No tears were shed as she was driven off in the back of a pickup truck.

But we did still have Theo, so when we moved into Cambridge, I immediately put in an electric fence. This, I hoped, would keep Theo safe. Only she never got the hang of that, or perhaps I am guilty of not properly following up with the fence training. It became a daily occurrence for Theo to run away past the fence and us to chase and retrieve her. Actually, she usually returned when she had had her fill of freedom, and occasionally neighbors would return her.

Theo ended up going to NYC with my older daughter, but when I moved to NYC myself, my daughter gave Theo back to me soon after. By then, Theo was fourteen and had become incontinent. The vet advised me to have her put to sleep.

Since I was living by myself in NYC, I once again thought that a dog would fill a void. I wanted a companion, so I again got excited about finding just the right dog. Chloe was a Shih Tzu and was affectionate, playful, and outgoing. She was my fourth dog.

When I would go away, I would ask my wonderful back elevator man, Arturo, if he would enjoy having her for the weekend. He and his children loved Chloe, and it took me awhile to notice that whenever they returned her to me, Chloe would leave a dump in the living room.

I was extremely slow to realize she vastly preferred Arturo's family to being with me. One day she climbed on top of a huge pile of papers on my desk and relieved herself there! When I moved from the East Side to the West Side, I wisely decided to give Chloe to Arturo. He was thrilled, and I know Chloe was as well.

My second marriage was to an art history professor. He was incredibly intelligent and was known world-wide as an expert in his field. I liked him and his son, and I was so lonely and eager for a relationship that I leaped into marriage with this man. I did not date him long enough to realize how depressed he was. At one time he told me that both of his grandfathers had com-mitted suicide!

The most difficult thing about my second husband was his tirades. They were so bad, and though I knew they were not really about me, that did not stop me from being frustrated and angry enough to once throw a vase across the room. One day a friend of mine visited and experienced one of Larry's outbursts, and afterward she mentioned she would never tolerate such a thing. Meanwhile, my mother's words rang in my head: "Give every relationship 75 percent."

Larry was a good man, but after four years I could see he was as unhappy as I was. When I asked whether he had been happy at all during the years we had been together, he said no. I got up from my chair, gave him a hug and a kiss on the cheek, and said, "Thank you for being so honest."

He then added, "But I never expected to be." I did not really know what that meant. Sadly, earlier in his life maybe he could not be who he truly was, and this likely led to his depression.

My third marriage was only a few years later. That husband worshipped me, putting me on a pedestal. Only later did I realize that that had a lot to do with my social status and money. However, I liked his courtly good manners and good humor. He had friends I liked, and I again found myself very lonely, so was thrilled at the prospect of a new chapter in my life.

This third husband was very friendly, had been fund-raising at Yale and at the Smithsonian, and I thought we could date happily. But he wanted us married, saying he could not go to Fisher's Island with a "girlfriend." He was seventy-four at the time. I stupidly gave in.

To give you a glimpse of my poor and impulsive judgment at that time, when he proposed (kneeling down when I was sitting on a bench on Fifth Avenue), I immediately said yes. We had known each other for about a year. That evening I called my four adult children, told them I was going to marry again, and then, one hour later, called them back and told them I would prefer to just go to the courthouse the next day to get married.

My youngest son was clerking for a judge downtown, so he met us and was our witness that next day. My youngest daughter was getting married in September, so I did not want to take away any limelight from her and was very influenced by my recent fiancé's eagerness.

This third husband wanted a dog, so we finally got him a Havanese because I had heard they were a lovely breed that did not shed. Her name was Raisin and she had given birth to six litters of puppies. She was a perfect lap dog and seemed very content being with a family who took such good care of her.

When I heard that Raisin had a sister named Gracie who was also ready to go to a forever home, I got her for myself. But just two weeks after her arrival, I gave her away to my ninety-year-old neighbor, another dog lover, who was thrilled. My third husband was part of the golf community where we lived, so when I decided to leave him, I also left that community, and that was why I gave this dog to my elderly neighbor. Once my daughter asked how much longer I would put up with being treated so poorly, I was able to pack up. She was the third person to tell me that I was putting up with "abuse."

Overall, our marriage lasted for six years. Like the second husband, the third one had rages and yelled at me. It was only after what my older daughter asked me that I decided to leave. He was eighty when I insisted we separate. A year later, he told me that he had known he was gay since he was sixteen.

I think you can now see why my children discouraged me so much when I told them I wanted to get a dog once I was settled in Rhinebeck. But I ignored them all and was determined to finally have a dog relationship that would make me happy. I was eager to have the companionship but somehow unable to look at my not-so-successful history of dog ownership. I also imagined that my four Rhinebeck grandchildren would adore my dog.

Three years ago, a friend came to visit from Guilford, Connecticut, and asked, "Why don't you have a dog?"

I responded, "Funny you should ask that. I just heard that my granddaughter might benefit from having a dog, but her parents aren't wanting one. I could get a little dog for her and for me."

"What kind of dog would you get?" my friend asked.

"A Havanese, because I know that breed is wonderful." Havanese are known for being circus dogs—intelligent, outgoing, and funny.

"Well, you are in luck because my neighbor breeds Havanese," she responded.

Within an hour of my friend's departure, I spoke to that neighbor. Apparently my requesting a black puppy limited my choices, but a date was set, and I was going to get my new furry friend that August.

My eldest grandchild named this dog Hector, and Hector was an adorable little puppy. Everyone in the neighborhood took an interest in him. I knew that training a dog was not something I was good at, so this time I hired a trainer—at great expense—who bullied me for months. Clearly, I was not good at being the assertive dog owner I needed to be. However, I was tenacious, so Hector and I dutifully went to our lessons in a big gym. I dreaded them, but I imagined this time I would have a beautifully trained dog.

Hector was such a dream that first year. I did not even mind too much walking him. But at his first birthday, he developed a truly fierce bark. For such a small, ten-pound dog, he sounded ferocious. The difficulty with this barking was that it drove me nuts. I have what is called an "exaggerated startle reflex," so with every bark I would jump a mile. I hated his barking and went back to the trainer, even trying two other trainers to see if they could get him to stop. Each time Hector spotted a squirrel or smelled or heard a dog, he would bark, startling me violently. One of the trainers urged me to order a gizmo from Amazon that would discourage the barking. I tried several different devices, but none of them worked.

Still, I held onto a dream that Hector would become a therapy dog. I had worked in hospitals as a volunteer in pediatrics and wanted to return to that, so I hired another woman who led classes for therapy dogs. This trainer said we could try but that Hector would have to be able to sit quietly on my front porch without barking while dogs and people went by. After the third lesson, we both realized it was hopeless. Hector was never going to be certified as a therapy dog.

Last year, a former nanny, Christina, had a tragic accident hit their family: her son was killed in a motorcycle accident. She asked if she could borrow Hector for comfort. She and her husband have a small dog named Rosie, and the two dogs got along because her family took care of Hector when I went away. One time when he was brought back to me, he cried for a long time after he was dropped off. He licked the side of his bed, and when I questioned Christina about why he started doing this, she suggested that it was because Hector would wake Rosie up by licking her ears. The next day Hector had an upset stomach and had to go to the vet.

I finally began to see that he, along his gut, was telling me something important. I also realized that I had to finally face myself as a woman who loves certain dogs but is not a genuine dog lover. I have never truly enjoyed walking any of my dogs, and the sudden loud barks were enough to put me in a bad mood every time.

However, there was also the important issue of "What will people think of me?" My neighbors had taken a lot of interest in Hector, and I did not want them to think badly of me. (Obviously, I have not told my dog history to many.) But it was a genuine concern for me as someone who is always trying to both please and, to some extent, appear better than I feel. What would they think of me if I gave away Hector?

Luckily for me, Hector showed me that he prefers living with Christina and her family to being without canine companionship at my house. So today, Hector has a new home, and I am extremely relieved to know it is what he wanted. My neighbors are kind and never made me feel bad about giving him away.

What have I learned? That much like my experience with owning a pet, I had unrealistic expectations of marriage and what it took to make the relationship successful for both parties.

I am thankful for my children and for my opportunities to leave marriages that were not working. I have learned that companionship does not have to come from a romantic relationship or a cute dog. I need to turn inward, and, in order to do that, I need to slow down.

Monica models moving at her own pace and advises me to leave more space between my activities. The best source of what I was looking for is coming from

Monica. She has shown me the unconditional motherly love I have always searched for.

Finally, I am not lonely. I have learned to listen to my feelings and can pause to notice how I am. I don't automatically rush in to try to meet someone else's needs, and I am more relaxed and able to see what my own feelings are. My own needs are taking priority.

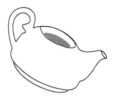

CHAPTER 5

Keeping Fear at Bay

Healing means, first of all, the creation of an empty but friendly space where those who suffer can tell their story to someone who can listen with real attention.

—Henry Nouwen

My friend Kathy just called from Los Angeles, and we talked for forty-five minutes. Just before hanging up, she said, "What was it about your energy that after one day in fourth grade, in spite of how you looked, I went home and told my parents that I had just met my new best friend?" When she referred to how I looked, she meant that I was covered with open sores and had started pulling out my already thinning hair.

Two years ago, I gave myself a seventy-fifth birthday party and invited about seventy female friends. What was so wonderful was that they ended up forming groups of women who got up and toasted me. The Spence School, where I was moved to from Town School for fourth grade, was a great new beginning for me. My friend Nancy told the group at my birthday lunch, which was held at the Cosmopolitan Club, that her mother liked me so much that she was jealous of me! I was so astounded to hear this, especially since I always did poorly in any academic endeavor and Nancy always got A's in every class.

It was a huge confidence builder to have different groups say I brought people together and created community. I realize now that this is what I am good at. I like meeting people, and now I want to use this gift to create something that makes me feel I have contributed to helping my community.

I have always been told that I have way more energy than many people of my age. Now I can see it a bit more clearly. I still enjoy jumping on the trampoline, and many of my contemporaries don't want to do much of any exercise. But my inquiry is about the *mystery* of energy. When I hear these flattering references to my past, I ponder something I was recently told: I need not try so hard; spirit would make it feel effortless.

But here I am this morning stressing over the simple task of writing a toast to Michael and then reading it aloud so it can be filmed and sent to him. I wrote one, but I don't think it was very good at all. So how do we acknowledge what our gifts are, stay grateful for them, and continue to be present? The important part is our expression—that we have done something with our best intention and effort, regardless of the reaction to it. We are meant to just be who we are, pray to be of use, and believe with our whole hearts that we are. I listen to those who tell us that we are bringing the light, and I sure pray this is the case in everything I do, even if it feels like a struggle or like what I do is not good enough. I pray my mind stays out of the way.

❋　❋　❋　❋　❋

My younger brother turns seventy years old today. He has lived a year longer than our father whose heart gave out at sixty-nine. This has led me to consider what helps us feel alive. What is it that we human beings need to feel connected to others?

Yesterday I met over Zoom with another trainee for the Healing Circles. We talked for an hour and were able to connect so easily, both of us feeling "called" to be hosts for the Healing Circles. This is a bond we discovered together, and I now feel connected to this oncology nurse in Iowa.

In his journal on the CaringBridge site, Michael Lerner explains this type of connection as a "heart journey." He says that when someone shares their story with us, they bring immense vitality, and he contends that when this vitality is gone, it could be a sign of being out of touch with one's heart source. In the final paragraph of his November 28th journal entry, he says, "I love being alive. I love it with the greatest intensity. I pray for many more years of this beautiful pulsating life. But when my time comes, I pray that I will have prepared myself for it. So that I can walk into Mystery and whatever the Mystery brings with it."

My memory goes back to a conversation I had many years ago with a friend from Chatham Hall, when I asked her, "Do you know what people mean when they say they 'love life'?"

She did not have an answer, and neither did I. Looking back from where I am now, I can see that I have been disconnected from my energy source for a major part of my life. But the way I feel now is exactly how Lerner describes his own vitality. I am working at staying connected, and one way is through sticking to my Qigong practice. Another way is by seriously learning how to host Healing Circles, and a third way is by writing about my experience.

So today I find myself sitting here in my kitchen, sipping my Irish Breakfast tea with oat milk, asking myself, "How can I be wanting to focus on this at 6:00 a.m. more than anything else today? Is it some

Guide leading me? Do I have an inner compass that leads me to the Source?"

How is it possible that this seventy-seven-year-old woman is the matured version of the rebellious teen-ager at Chatham Hall? That girl who was unwilling to kneel or sing in chapel? Prayer seemed ridiculous, and now I want to pray all day long.

I have also never enjoyed puzzles of any kind, but now all I want is to be able to put together some fragments of understanding. I wish to help my grand-children better understand what has taken me so many decades to discover. Of course, I do realize that this is not something you just read and get. But I still want to make the effort for myself and plant seeds for them.

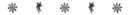

I have been talking with many people and am so impressed by how nourishing some of my conversations are. One topic of interest to me is nonviolent communi-cation. It is so important to me, I now realize, because I want to be an effective host of Healing Circles.

I also learned from Michael Lerner's CaringBridge journal about Sharon Ellison and her description of powerful non-defensive communication, or PNDC™. Her website states that PNDC is "a revolutionary para-digm that allows us to protect ourselves without getting defensive and to achieve our goals without resorting to power struggle. With this model, we can simultaneously be direct and honest as well as open and transparent, thereby increasing our integrity without losing spontaneity. In the process, we can enhance our own creativity and success, while prompting others to have greater respect and care for us. The surprise is that we can have far more power, rather than less."[4]

All these ideas are swirling inside of me this morning as the rain pounds down. My nineteen-year-old granddaughter is sitting next to me at my kitchen island with her computer. I recognize each stage of life has its joys and struggles, and today I am opening myself up to the curiosities today brings—without judgment.

❋　❦　❋　❦　❋

Years ago, in a conversation with my friend and writing teacher Marta, she casually commented that I live an "overly populated life," which struck me as a perfect title for a writing subject. I would not want to make it too serious or spend too much time on it, so I will just quickly mention why that struck a nerve in a good way.

When my father got custody of us, he had no idea how to discipline children. He allowed my brothers to

---

4. "What is PNDC," Powerful Non-Defensive Communication (PNDC), accessed June 3, 2022, https://www.pndc.com/about/.

wrestle, tackle, and pummel me whenever they got the urge. My father never, that I can remember, told them to stop. Maybe Daddy did not want to incite a grand mal seizure in my brother, who knows. My stepmother came along when I was six, and she and Daddy had four more children, two years apart. This second litter was less of a problem because they always had nannies who took care of them. But I had a lot of siblings. I remember once being asked how many siblings I had, and I answered, "Too many," appalled it had popped out of my mouth!

My father was on the board of the Experiment in International Living, which was a program for adolescents to experience living abroad in another culture. (It is now called World Learning.) He loved having people stay with us in our duplex apartment in NYC. There were strangers at breakfast frequently, and they hung around a lot. Cousins of my father's also came to stay from Italy and from Holland, and they were sometimes in residence for months at a time.

I think this influenced me, because this "welcoming home" has continued to be a value of mine. In my adult life, I took on this role in my family by being the initiator of hospitality. I think this also maybe created my pattern of being busy and never really feeling grounded. My self-soothing strategy for this was to make friends at school. Fortunately, I eventually made it to the all-girls Spence School in fourth grade. I was told not to return to the progressive, co-ed Town School because there I kept getting in fights with the boys during recess. That school recommended psychiatric help, but my father told me he said no to this suggestion for fear my mother would make fun of me.

Once I got to the Spence School, I made close friends, which enabled me to get the attention I craved. What I can see in hindsight is that it also partially filled the void of motherly love. Ever since that fourth-grade year, I have been collecting female friends who have stayed with me, and I feel I might not have survived without them.

At a later period in my life, I moved eight times in twelve years, and that meant I rushed to make friends in each new community. This was a reasonably successful strategy, but it meant I was perpetually on the go. Now that COVID-19 has arrived, I am delighted to slow down, but my schedule is still pretty full. In fact, I often double-book friends coming over to visit on my back porch because my memory is slipping almost as rapidly as one day rolls into the next week. Now I just say, "Please just text me to see if it is a good time."

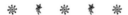

Here I am in my reading room, glad to have twenty minutes in which to write about my resume. I do have one, although I have not looked at it in probably a full decade. I am lucky, because as a social worker I have been able to do what I most enjoy even without an actual job.

Now that I am in this pandemic chapter, I feel as though I can ignore my resume completely. I am experiencing a kind of freedom that is new and am discovering its preciousness. I no longer have to abide by others' desires for how I use my time. I did not realize how much I was meeting others' expectations until these past months.

These days, I use my energy primarily to keep fear at bay. The media is assaulting us, and I am surprised by how quickly I turn off the mainstream media. I guess my resume, if it were based on my mind and behavior, would show my inner rebel. I admit to having never been a rule follower, but now I am looked at as a person who questions "authority." We are told to wear masks, but if we read statements from doctors other than the ones we are told to admire, we hear contrary opinions.

Since my resume has never claimed any proficiency in debating, I step out of that arena. I wait for others to form their committees and trust that they will bring sense to the many rule followers. Yes, I refuse to argue because I am not well informed, nor do I have any proficiency in logical debate. I simply appreciate that there are like-minded souls with whom I can converse on this subject.

Keeping my neighbors from discussing their fear of going into CVS or grocery stores is requiring too much of my energy. I don't want to engage in swapping stories about people who have been seen not wearing masks. I want to use my energy to read from and listen to the people who are lifting my spirits, not those who put a pin into my balloon of optimism.

My balloon is simply made up of the belief that, in time, good will win over evil. I think we will discover a great deal we were ignorant of, but each of us will deal with it as best we can. So, I will keep on hoping that we will not hurt one another during this time of such political craziness. May each of us realize how much we can influence one another.

❋　❦　❋　❦　❋

Many years ago, my brother Beek told me a story about an evening a few months prior when he was in our place in South Carolina with our younger siblings. After he started summarizing what had transpired, I stopped him and said, "I was there, Beek. Why are you acting as if I wasn't?"

He argued with me, claiming I could not have been there. I reminded him that, contrary to his lousy memory, I *was* there. This made me so angry because it was common for me to feel that I was both unseen and unheard.

All this just feels important this morning as I try to focus on how to tell my own story. I have been writing this memoir for about a year now and have kept journals for decades. My writing teacher says I am a writer, but I still somehow question it. My low self-esteem has been a major issue all my life.

Had I been unconsciously seeking healing before I was intentionally seeking it? Now that I am consciously discovering myself, I believe that I was. In so many ways, I was trying to fill these holes I unconsciously knew existed.

※　❋　※　❋　※

The day of my son Michael's fiftieth birthday was one of revelation for me. Two days before, I had impulsively decided to send "favors" out by UPS so that I could be there in spirit since I was not invited to be there in person.

Three of my four children were getting together to celebrate. I had heard the celebration was to be outdoors and socially distant so their favorite musician, Will Oldham, could play for them. What fun I had selecting lovely, warm, and handsome gloves for my family.

When I got home from purchasing the gloves, I added to the gifts some new tea from India. It was loose-leaf tea, so I added a little container to put on the teapot along with the tea. I also put in two new packages of birthday napkins, one set with blue checks, and a plastic blue-and-white checkered picnic table-cloth. It was a rather whimsical collection, and I was aware of how it was typical of me to assemble such an odd assortment.

I absolutely loved every part of putting it all together. I enjoyed using only old ribbons and tissue paper, picking the favorite colors of the recipients, finding the perfect card for each of them, and writing a personalized note in each one. Carefully, I slipped the notes under the ribbon so that each person would get the right gift. I was really thrilled, and when I put the lid on, I felt so happy. It would be a surprise, although I did write Michael ahead of time to have him watch for it. I wanted him to understand the reason for his blue-and-white theme was that, fifty years ago, I was thrilled to have given birth to a boy! I told Michael how I dressed my son in blue since my older daughter did not have much blue in her wardrobe. Sending this blue-checkered box full of thoughtful gifts made me so happy. Birthdays were always special to me. When the four children were little, I always gave each child an early birthday gift at breakfast.

I carefully carried the box full of gifts to my car and then into UPS, where, to my absolute horror, I was told it would cost over $250 to ship! I debated, but I thought to myself, "I am lucky to be able to do this, and at least the gifts will arrive on the exact day" and handed over my credit card.

The next morning, I got a call from Michael thanking me. When he said he was delighted with the two pairs of gloves, I said, "No, Michael, one pair is for Nathaniel. Didn't you see the card?"

"Oh no," he said. "I'm afraid the contents were all messed up. There weren't any cards, and the wrappings were all torn off." My disappointment was enormous, but I could not talk at that moment and did not say much.

Upon reflection, I think the universe somehow made that checkered blue box into a symbol. Who knows how it got smashed, but it most certainly helped me understand a new way of looking at my role as a parent to adult children. They chose not to include me, but I prefer not to be present if I am not wanted. I have a life and now have the inner strength to stand alone. The smashed box was a physical example of my squished dream. I am still chewing on the meaning of this disappointment.

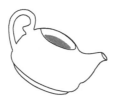

CHAPTER 6

Heading Toward
a Clean Slate

*True belonging doesn't require you to change
who you are; it requires you to be who you are.*

—Brené Brown

With my fourth pregnancy, I was certain that I would try again for natural childbirth. And I succeeded. When the obstetrician reached to help pull my baby Nathaniel out, he told me that although the umbilical cord was wrapped twice around Nathaniel's neck, it was loose and had not caused any difficulty for this infant boy. From that moment on, I knew how fortunate I was.

Only a few minutes later, the doctor explained that he would now need to medicate me in order to tie my tubes! I had not realized that this would be a hard follow-up to the excitement of Nathaniel's birth, but I was not about to object. I also did not know that a student would be performing the procedure, not the doctor himself. (Now, in all fairness, the doctor may have asked if this was okay, and I would not have objected if he did ask me.) But the problem came later.

After a day or two in the hospital, I was to go home with Nathaniel. I remember being at the elevator in a wheelchair and the nurse holding my baby, when I suddenly felt my incision open up and blood spill out all over my pants. I was rushed up to the operating room, and thankfully the problem was resolved surgically. However, I was told it necessitated a few more days and nights in the hospital. The good news was, I still got to breastfeed my baby and was in a very good mood. I now had my complete family. I knew I was blessed to have two boys and two girls, all under the age of six.

I, too, had been a fourth child, albeit an unwanted one, and I was determined to have a very much wanted final child. One of my most favorite happy memories is the time I danced at the Lincoln Nursery School party with infant Nathaniel strapped onto my front, held securely as his parents waltzed. As the music from *My Fair Lady* played, I felt such joy that I truly felt

I could have danced all night. Nathaniel was only a few weeks old, and that memory has been with me now for nearly five decades.

※　❋　※　❋　※

Do you know the feeling of having nothing to say and wondering how you can possibly be interested in anything? This is how I have felt many times when I am in a social situation and am exhausted. It took me years to realize that is what made me feel as though the blackboard of my mind had been erased.

An image I shared with others when it happened is when I was at a dinner party once and the man next to me got so bored that he pulled out his cell phone and just focused on that. This would not have bothered me as much as it did, except for the fact that our host was across the table and took this in. She had invited me as her guest and had carefully seated us next to each other. Sadly, I was a flop at this fundraising dinner.

Now, during this Coronavirus time, I have a similar image that perplexes me. It is still on my mind's blackboard, but now my mind has been washed clean. No more faint chalk marks or blurry, old writing; it is simply erased. A wet sponge has been put to the blackboard of my mind, and it is both refreshing and soothing.

I cry often, but my vulnerability makes me aware of being alive. When I am awake at night for several hours,

I can feel my body against the sheets and be aware of the comfort of lying still. I then wish all beings could be so relaxed.

What goes on in my mind are all the things I want to do the next day. I realize, for example, that my children's father is celebrating his eightieth birthday on November 9th. I want to send him a card, but I realize there is not time for that, so I will email him instead. Clearly these are not important thoughts, but they please me. They are small things, but even imagining my morning routine of making tea gives me a sense of wanting to get up the next day. This is different from during pre-Coronavirus times. I was more pressured then than I feel now. My brain was constantly going, and I slipped into feeling overwhelmed way more than enjoying relaxation.

There are peculiarities of my mind that I am more conscious of these days. When I am enjoying something a lot, it is hard for me to stay with it to enjoy it all the way through. I impulsively want to share it with others. For example, when I was listening to the interview with Michael Tilson Thomas on PBS called "American Masters," I instantly realized that I wanted my four children to hear it. But I was able to stop myself from immediately reaching for my phone and texting them.

What is this impulse to give my pleasure away to someone else? I wonder whether it is my effort to be in control. Or am I hoping for an exchange of gratitude? I just like the fact that my awareness is helping me change. Is it possible that my Qigong practice is helping bring about more clarity? I do know that I am far more aware of the people I wish to keep close and care less than I used to about remaining connected to so many people. Since learning about Dr. Gabor Maté's work, I have wondered whether this is a habit I developed to survive my early childhood. Now I see that it was a technique that helped me get some of my needs met.

In this strange time, I have the opportunity to look at who I have turned into. I am amused by what has stayed and what is slipping away. For example, I am questioning things I never did before, and they are not things that other people believe. Am I possibly becoming more confident in my questioning? I like to hope that I am. I am starting to write a few sentences on the blackboard of my new, uncluttered mind. One could surmise that perhaps I am beginning to trust my curiosity and allow my uncertainty to be a constant.

My dear friend Holly just called me tonight to tell me that she is being taken in an ambulance tomorrow morning to the hospital to see if there is anything that can be done. Two days ago she was diagnosed with cancerous tumors on her spine as well as a broken spine. It is so serious that if she moves the wrong way, she will be completely paralyzed!

Holly called me to say what a good friend I have been and that I listen in a way quite different from other friends. She has been in a quandary about whether to go get this other opinion, but she felt it was either do nothing and wait to die or find out that maybe there is a chance that it is not as dire as it seems today.

Last fall, Holly and I helped our mutual friend Arvia sell apples. We had taken advantage of Arvia's swimming pool over the summer, so volunteering to help sell apples from her glorious orchard was a way to show our gratitude. Holly and I sat near the beautiful apple trees and greeted each of the cars that drove up. Some of them had children inside, but many did not. We offered the guests bags to purchase for $10 or $20 and supplied them with a picker, a long pole that makes reaching for the apples way up high a little easier.

Holly and I took turns with the greetings and then sat back down to talk. I was amazed to discover that being outdoors without anything to do other than this simple taking of money and providing the pickers was so conducive to intimate conversation. It was not too surprising, however, since when we would swim, Holly and I would stand in the shallow part of the pool and talk for hours. I began to become aware of being more present.

But today, with news of my friend's condition, my body feels heavy, my voice sounds funny to me, and my body has been sort of shaking. I have not cried yet, but hopefully I will do that when I get into bed tonight.

Holly and I met when we took the same class at Bard College. It was an intriguing course called "Living an Undefended Life." We both liked the teacher, and that was where we became friends. What continues to delight me is the way friendships grow. Ours deepened quite quickly because of our going to Arvia's for walks as well as to swim. We found it easy to talk with one another; I would recount things that I had done, and she always seemed to understand. She told me a lot about her years in Dayton, Ohio, and about her children. We agreed a lot about some of the cultural norms of the time when we were raising our children and agreed we may have fallen into some of the same patterns.

This time of "letting go" in life sure is difficult. Being at the front of a family with four kids, I got used to being center stage. Now I am in the back row and cannot even see what is happening on the stage! I am adjusting to the role of grandmother and am trying to just let go of my no-longer-applicable expectations.

What interests me now is that which is very immediate, and day-to-day is all I can do. I know that my memory is only getting worse, but so are my friends' memories, and during this weird time we have trouble knowing what month it is some days.

What I know for sure is that Holly is a friend who understands me and loves me, and I love her dearly. What I can focus on now is just being here for her as long as I can be.

*   *   *   *   *

If I could change one thing about my body, it would be to accept it without judgment and know that it is trying to tell me something when it brings me discomfort. My skin is the issue, and I do realize now, after seven decades of eczema, that I need to listen to the outbreaks.

The first two times Winifred gave me treatments, she insisted on giving them to me for free so that I could see if they had any benefits for me. Well, let me tell you, Winifred warned me that there would be a change as soon as she moved my energy. She told me, "It will stir up your system, so your skin and your tummy will react. The purpose is to get energy moving. When energy is stagnant, it isn't good, and symptoms will develop. So, you need to be okay with that. Are you?"

I said I was, but I later wondered why I did not wait a week so that I would not be in an unsettled state when my son and his wife arrived with their two boys. The plans these past three months have changed almost as rapidly as they have been made.

When my skin erupted so ferociously that I had blood back on my sheets like I did as a child, I was miserable both physically and mentally. Psychologically I was back to being ten years old, and although this time I did not pull my hair out (literally), I was so sad and in such pain with my rash all over my face and chest, and my ears were raw with the scratching in my sleep. I will not linger on this, but suffice it to say, I questioned my judgment about doing this when I had company coming. I thought I had been, as usual, a bit impulsive and, frankly, stupid. But, being an excellent rationalizer, I decided it was not such a bad idea after all. They have now seen what their Nonnie looks like during an outbreak.

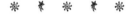

Eva was my nanny from the time I was about five until my stepmother sent her away. I loved her very much and decided to write her a letter, although she will likely never read it:

Dearest Eva,

You were the person I loved more than anyone. I stopped believing in God after you left, Eva. Now I am an old lady remembering how you planted the seeds that have finally blossomed.

It is a gloomy day, and I feel terrible this afternoon. It is the beginning of a new year, but I am disconnected and extremely sad. I will allow myself to ramble in hopes of arriving at something. My purpose is to thank you. Amazingly, I believe not only in life after death but in our ability to be guided.

Whether you are one of the helpers who have been with me my whole life, maybe I will never know, but what I do know is that I am grateful for the ability to sit here in my living room in Rhinebeck with the fire going, a cup of tea next to me, and the desire to write about how I now look at the world.

Just a few weeks ago I read Into the Magic Shop *by James Doty, MD. Then I listened to Bruce Lipton, MD talking about how our thoughts shape our reality. I have been reading about these ideas for some time, but it was not until I could allow myself to be vulnerable to what others might say that I could actually speak "my truth" and felt ready to write to you.*

You not only always treated me with kindness and love, but also never scolded me or told me to "stop scratching" my eczema! You knew what I felt like, inside and out, and you gave me empathy. I did not know then that your way of treating me canceled out all the shame I felt. My older brothers were not able to provide any comfort, and, sadly, neither were either of my parents or stepparents. You, alone, were the person who saw me, listened to me, and put salve on my emotional as well as my physical wounds.

How can I not remember you teaching me to pray? You gave me words and images, and I loved saying them with you. But after you left, I let all that fall away. What you did not know was that I carried your love with me.

I truly believe it is because of you that I have been able to trust people and form strong relationships. I have had some rocky times, especially because I had repercussions from the time before I met you. In the past year, I have been interested in the work of two psychiatrists who are roughly my age. They are Bessel van der Kolk and Gabor Maté, both experts in early childhood trauma. What I have pieced together are fragments. Out of these I have made a story about why I am the way I am and why Mummy became an alcoholic.

While Daddy fought hard to keep the marriage, Mummy was really adamant about the divorce she requested just after my birth. Based on what I have learned, Mummy most likely had been drinking heavily for some time. I don't know the extent of that and am sad that so much is murky, but telling you what I know makes me feel better. The divorce happened and Daddy got custody. I was told that Mummy's alcoholism was a factor, and I now think she probably had been sexually abused as a child. I feel no need to go into why I came to this conclusion, but part of it is through my friendship with Mummy's niece who has shared things with me I did not know before.

It is only now, in 2021, that we are facing the extent of how many children are sexually abused. What I now realize is that the shame is devastating. I think Mummy drank because of some completely unconscious need to cover up her feelings.

I want to tell you why I feel so indebted to you and somehow allow myself to write about my life in what may seem to be a superficial manner. I don't think of myself as an intellectual, but I do see that what really interests me is relationships. I have spent years feigning interest in many things such as art and music, but it really turns out to be watching movies and reading books about relationships that captures my attention.

You gave me the attention I so craved, dear Eva, and it did so much to bolster my sense of self. But what I have learned is that when that brain circuitry does not get developed as it should when one is an infant, that person has difficulty knowing what their inner self really wants. I am still sorting this out but do think my difficulty in choosing husbands who would really nurture me and care for me was partly due to this insufficiency.

The part that is of particular interest has to do with brain development. When I was an infant, certainly Mummy was stressed. She told me many times in the years that followed that she had never wanted me, and that John, the eldest of my three brothers, was the only child she ever wanted! I accepted this, but I believe that as an infant I may have given up fully expressing my needs in order to get my attachment secured with Mummy. The result, as I try to comprehend what Dr. Gabor Maté says, is that the circuitry of my brain did not develop as it would have if I had been emotionally secure. As you well know, I broke out with severe eczema when I was only a few months old. I believe my body was expressing what I was feeling, and I had no control over any of it. But you were there for me.

At all times in school, I was unable to really pay attention. A lot of it was due to physical discomfort from the incessant itching and scratching of my eczema, but I also had, as it turns out, severe learning disabilities. I, of course, concluded that I was stupid.

This is where Maté's work and research are particularly helpful to me. Any child who cannot do the work that academic settings provide makes this negative self-judgment. Once I decided it would not do me any good to study, I did not really try. Instead, I tried to get the attention I craved by acting out. This was a constant behavior, yet no one ever tried to help me look at it and understand what was going on. So, it continued right into high school.

Then there was college. I went to three different ones and finally came away with a degree in general studies from Columbia University. By then, I was married and teaching at the Dalton School. But I cannot go this slowly through my many decades. What I want to say is that your introduction to a spiritual side of me is what has sustained me.

I went on to do clinical pastoral education twice. My education came mostly after college, and although I managed to secure two master's degrees, the real learning was in internships and workshops. The thread of being interested in finding God was there. I was led to do hospice work for three years and got the social work degree as well as one in counseling and psychology. I have always been seeking answers.

Thank you, dear Eva, for giving me a way to go forward after you left. I am grateful to you for helping me turn to God.

You have my deepest love always,
Alexandra

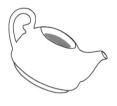

CHAPTER 7

Shifting from Contentment to Joy

Some people think they are in community, but they are only in proximity. True community requires commitment and openness. It is a willingness to extend yourself to encounter and know the other.

—David Spangler

I have jokingly referred to myself as "The Tea Lady of Rhinebeck" because I easily invite people over and enjoy having them be relaxed in my comfortable house. I have noticed that my way of entertaining has shifted. I still like having strangers someone has suggested

I meet come over for tea, but I am more selective and always keep the group small.

Over a year ago, I attempted to bring some neighbors together to meet a newcomer to the area. It was, from my point of view, a disaster. First of all, I made the preparations way more complicated than they needed to be. I was aware of the immense fear of COVID, so I had separate little plates of cookies in several places on my front porch. Then there was the honey, the sugar cube, the pitchers of both dairy and nondairy creamers, the caffeinated pot of tea, and the herbal teapot. I had not thought that people would want iced tea; after all, though it was a hot and humid day, it was also overcast.

The awkwardness of the conversation was something I did not anticipate either. I have rarely found the company so stiff, and because three of us are quite deaf and socially distanced, it was even more so. Worst of all was the mask issue. My friend, who was ninety-two years old at the time, did not wear one and was clearly looked at with judgment by another. The newcomer, the reason for the party, was eighty-three and had just been diagnosed with Lyme disease that day, so she was in an unusually distraught state. When she rambled about the diagnosis, none of us could follow her. I attempted to be sympathetic but was distracted by playing host.

Suddenly, I was asked whether I had any iced tea and excused myself to the kitchen. When I went inside to arrange the glasses and get the herbal and caffeinated iced tea, I realized what a relief it was to come inside—and it was not just the air conditioning! My tea party was not working out as I had hoped, and I decided in that moment that I certainly was not going to do it again.

A few minutes after I reappeared on the porch, one of my neighbors instructed us that we should all get home soon because of the arriving black clouds and impending storm. This was not in the forecast, and the rest of us did not see the ominous black clouds she spoke of. Frankly, the only black cloud was her, and with her proclamation we all felt dismissed. Dutifully, the other ladies all left.

It was horribly unpleasant with the stifling heat, COVID rearrangements, my discomfort and overdoing, and the general awkwardness of conversation and attitudes on my porch that day. Maybe I will give up the title of "The Tea Lady of Rhinebeck" and therefore find more peace. I have learned to have fewer people to tea and to keep it simple.

❊　❦　❊　❦　❊

The woman I described as "the newcomer" has since become a friend. We take Friday morning walks together and enjoy going slow-paced through our neighborhood. Yesterday I managed to make my goal of five thousand steps. My app worked for both of us, so she was delighted when I told her that she, too, had made that goal.

I am curious about what made our walks so fun. The first week we wound up on my back porch, and she was clearly amazed that she was back there with me. She said, "I don't know why you are willing to keep coming back. I have been so remiss. I forget to return calls and somehow you are always here." I was touched.

I have also learned that I need companionship to guarantee that I will get a walk in. She and I have shared a few stories, and one in particular has cemented our friendship for me. A few weeks back I accepted her invitation for tea. We sat on her screened-in porch in the pouring rain. She admired my bright blue slicker and black hat and commented on my attire generally: "You have such style, Alexandra."

Her statement reminded me of a stranger I had met a few years back at a Vassar College gathering. I had asked a very attractive elderly woman if she would like to share a bagel with me, as we were all newcomers. She smiled brightly and said she would be delighted to. We sat and sipped our tea together, and when I told her I really liked her outfit, she replied, "Well, thank you. I am one of those people who can't answer the door without my earrings on."

I knew in that moment I met a kindred spirit. Though I never saw that woman again, I have always remem-bered that comment. I now feel compelled to make an effort to look the best I can, no matter what. After my morning shower, for example, I put on cologne and a tinted moisturizer and fix my hair carefully, even though it is still short.

What is adorable about this neighbor whom I have befriended is not only her compliments about my clothes but also her very long description of why she likes her new home. She once turned to me and said, "Oh dear! While I was making our tea, before you arrived, I promised myself I wouldn't monopolize the conversation. I told myself, 'Let Alexandra speak' and yet, look what I did."

I laughed and responded, "That is a riot, because on my walk over here, I told myself, 'Alexandra, please remember to let your friend talk. You don't need to tell her every thought you have had in the last day.'" We chuckled, and our friendship was cemented.

❊ ❦ ❊ ❦ ❊

I never managed to keep track of all the psychotherapists I sought help from, but there were many. One of the most important was Dr. Putnam. He was a Jungian and helped me by interpreting my dreams. He said he was merely the midwife of my new insights, and I was grateful for his asking me about why I needed to keep so busy. But despite this work, I never really got more than a whiff of what the driving force of my life was.

I knew there was a powerful engine behind my high energy and that there was a reason for the excessive doing, doing, and more doing.

I found it easy to get as far as understanding that both of my parents approved of getting things done. My oldest brother is an excellent example of our childhood conditioning. He routinely double-books lunches so he can fit more people into his day. He, like me, wants both attention and praise, a sort of validation for having a reason to be on this planet.

I suppose we might both claim to truly enjoy all these companions without being able to really be present with them. We try and can sometimes focus, but certainly the need for a sense that we are liked and appreciated is stronger than our truly taking in what the person has offered us with their presence.

What might best convey my frantic racing through life is to describe what I see as the Florida chapter of my life. I was with my third husband, who took me for a first visit to a golf community called Mt. Lake, an hour south of Orlando. It did not take long for me to love the climate and the nice folks from all over the US who all shared the polite customs of good manners that I had been raised to appreciate. I liked many of the golf and bridge lovers because they were so nice to me. But it took less than a month or two for me to see that the real potential friends would be the ones I met by volunteering in the local public school.

The head of the school, Donna Dunson, and I became friends quickly. One day, I asked if we could use my wonderful friendships from the Spence School to help her transform her high school. Donna suggested I might start a speaker series as a part of that initiative. To my delight, the friends I invited down to Florida to give talks to the high school students all accepted. There were others I asked from my pool of friends, and they, too, agreed to come. Although I never paid these friends, they all came and gave wonderful talks; some spoke to two hundred students and others to fifteen hundred. I was in heaven making these arrangements and also felt the need to entertain and house these friends. This meant a great deal of rushing about to figure out meals, tours, and whatever I needed to do to show them my appreciation. It all actually went very well, and by the time I left I had introduced thirty-two different speakers to the high school in three years.

I kept track of all the overnight guests my third husband, Tim and I had, and in one four-month season we had forty-three friends stay! This gives you an idea of how busy I kept myself. Donna insisted on naming the school initiative "Alexandra's Speakers Series," which has continued, and I'm proud to have launched it. Looking back at it all, I savor the moments but mercifully no longer feel compelled to be quite that consumed with busyness.

❋ ❦ ❋ ❦ ❋

How else can I show you how busy I used to keep myself? If I show you my calendar, you may be impressed by the number of scribbles on each page, but even now my calendar looks pretty full. I wonder if I am partly kidding myself when I brag about how much quieter my life is. I guess I am still trying to show my world that what I do is of value. Actually, I am still trying to believe I have a contribution to make. If I can be myself and trust that that is sufficient, then I am content.

I am not pleased that this tendency is still evident, but then the saying "You can't turn an ocean liner around on a dime" comes back to remind me of my friend's sympathetic response to the sluggishness of my slowing down. You see, I think I am trying to prove to those who may care that I am no longer trying to distract myself from all that is in the way of the peace I am still striving for.

I really do now experience times of feeling peaceful, and that is a step forward. Let's give you a glimpse of this morning: I woke at 4:00 a.m. and decided to listen to my Audible book, so I put my phone on my pillow and turned on *Medical Medium* by Anthony William. So far, I have listened to approximately four of the twenty-two hours of content.

After I got up at 6:00 a.m. and made tea, I showered and dressed, wrote in my journal, and checked my email; then I did Qigong with Master Lu. At 8:50 a.m., I helped take a friend to get new tires and then had a long talk with my older son. I then spent time talking to a friend who helped me make some personal arrangements that are even better than I was expecting. That is another value of great relationships!

These past few days have been busy with conversations, but I did decide to announce to two of my friends that I no longer wish to have our regular phone hours on FaceTime. I realize that, unlike how I used to feel, being required to sit and talk with even these dear friends is rather like a noose around my neck. Instead, I want the freedom to choose when and if that is what I want to do, not to have it be an appointment.

To my surprise, both friends were understanding and told me they did not mind that I am giving myself room to be more spontaneous. I really am trying to clear my calendar of obligations. I have a few classes, but not many now, and I believe I have made some progress. I used to have one appointment after another all day every day. Now it is just a few per day.

The habit of being busy is still there, but when I discover I can just relax and look at one of my books, it is a good feeling. I have a big pile of books now that I have liked, and I am just starting to label them. I use sticky notes to write why I particularly liked the book and ask myself what I got out of it.

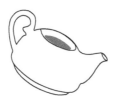

CHAPTER 8

Cleaning House

Let yourself be silently drawn by the strange
pull of what you really love. It will not
lead you astray.

—Rumi

The first time I saw Rob Wergin was in the Netflix documentary *Heal*. Later, when I heard he was going to give a workshop at Omega, the conference center near me here in Rhinebeck, I decided to register. When a friend in Boston heard I planned to attend, she offered to "check him out for me" as he was also presenting in Boston. After seeing him locally, she reported back to me that she thought it was a "cult." I took my name off the list for that gathering.

However, on the Saturday afternoon of Wergin's workshop in Rhinebeck, I suddenly realized I wanted to check him out for myself. So, I asked a neighbor who had never been to Omega if she would like to come along. I did not explain that I was there to stalk this man who was leading a workshop.

To my amazement, when we walked up to Omega's café level, there was Wergin talking with two women. I led my friend to an adjacent table and attempted to eavesdrop but did not have a lot of success. When Wergin got up, I explained to my friend that I was going to follow him and would be back shortly. To my delight, I found that he was heading into the bookstore next door. This made it easy for me to approach him, and so I did.

Wergin struck me as immediately likable, and he invited me to come to his free healing workshop at 7:00 p.m. After telling him I would be there, I drove the fifteen minutes back to my friend's house, quickly returned, and arrived just in time for the workshop.

I felt very pleased when Wergin recognized me and chose me to come up for a healing session in front of the group of 125 people sitting in a semicircle around him. The other people who were picked to demonstrate his healing were from France and Taiwan. We were asked to say what our presenting problem was in a few sentences. I said, "My skin and gut issues have been with me all my life."

Putting his hands on my front and back, Wergin announced, "You have already had a lot of healing," which I was fascinated by. He had not told anyone else that, and when he began to direct energy toward my body, mind, and spirit, I felt a gentle vibration.

The three people who had preceded me had fallen over into the arms of the helpers because of the strength of the vibrations they felt. Wergin always has helpers up on the stage to catch the people who come in for his healing, as many do fall from the forcefulness of the vibration from him. My experience was gentle, and the contrast with others was amazing to me.

After Wergin performed that healing on me, my eczema became decidedly much worse. I knew that alternative healing often causes a "healing crisis," so I prayed this was simply a result of whatever he had done. Eventually my eczema improved, so I decided to sign up for his next October workshop at Omega. I believed that healing had occurred but understood this phase was simply a part of the process. Wergin emphasized the importance of realizing the eczema was on its way out of my system, a thought that has been reassuring me long after his workshop.

Nevertheless, I was surprised by how bad my skin was a week later. The first thing Wergin had asked the 125 of us was, "How many of you found that your symptoms got worse before this workshop?" Many hands flew up, and Rob said that he did not know why this usually happened but that it always did.

Once again, I was very fortunate to be chosen to have a healing session in front of the group. As Wergin explained, the healing he demonstrates provides everyone in the room with healing energy. He is quick to explain that he has no idea why he has been given the power to be a conduit for healing energy. In fact, he told our group a short summary of his own story: When he was a little boy, he had the power to heal animals. His parents were "religious" and did not like that he had this ability, so he went on to a career path that his parents liked. In fact, he became the CEO of a successful corporation and made millions of dollars. Then in the 1980s, he lost everything and tried to commit suicide.

Wergin told us that he later heard a voice that said, "Go back and do what you did as a child. This time heal people as they are in great need of healing." He has been doing that ever since. Rob is kind, compassionate, full of good humor, and totally believable. Ever since he started using his gift, he has filled two workshops a year, always with over a hundred people. I went home full of optimism, although he warned us that our symptoms might get a lot worse before they got better. Mine did. However, he also emphasized that even when they return or worsen, we must realize that they are on their way out.

The year before this I had another experience of healing. I was in agony with a red rash all over my body that I had had for two months. I kept believing that the condition would improve, but it sure was taking a long time. It was the week before Christmas, and I had gone to a new alternative place of healing called the Bio Med Center in Providence, Rhode Island. I was there for five days of treatments and came away a devoted fan of this amazing place.

What I had not anticipated was the huge healing crisis that occurred after the visit. The treatments were over on a Friday, and I had planned a day of celebration for my seventy-fifth birthday on that Saturday, December 22, 2019. But by late afternoon on Friday, I felt as though I was coming down with a terrible flu and could no longer do anything but get in my car and drive home.

Then came two solid months of real physical agony, which naturally also made me depressed. I could not sleep because the intense itching was so uncomfortable. I would get up, take off my pajama top, and rub my back against the sharp edge of the wall or try to reach my back with my hairbrush, but it was not very good at relieving the itching. Sometimes I took a shower just to get another feeling on my skin. During the day I only wore white turtlenecks that felt soft on my skin and could be bleached to get out the blood stains. I felt terribly self-conscious because the splotches of red were obvious and people did not want to mention it or even ask how I was doing. I sometimes brought it up, but the explanation is difficult to put into a few sentences.

I was immensely relieved to find others on the internet who were trying to get off cortisone and had a community on Facebook, but I was not quite there yet. I just read the posts and listened to the videos of these fellow sufferers.

Ultimately, I discovered that I was suffering from red skin syndrome, a condition that those who overuse cortisone frequently suffer from. I knew it was not the eczema that I had had all my life, but I had never heard of this. Foolishly, I had allowed my connection to the National Eczema Association lapse. If I had read their newsletter, I would have known about this condition.

Three months after my first marriage, my skin had another eruption. But I was used to them, and so was startled when my father-in-law answered my question about which major should I choose (English or History) with the statement "You know, Alexandra, I think your skin condition has to be your top priority now."

I was startled because I was used to my erratic skin. I took his comment seriously and the new dermatologist put me into New York University Hospital for a solid month. That was in 1966 and cortisone was tried on me during that hospital stay, and I had injections, then pills, then strong creams.

Given that the cortisone hid the symptoms, I became addicted to using the creams. I was also oblivious to the connections between my gut and my skin. I finally found a gastroenterologist in 2016 after an explosive diarrhea attack on the street in NYC. This occurred on the day I was to fly to Tel Aviv with friends from Auburn Seminary.

When I returned, I dealt with my gut and skin by turning to both Western medicine and to complementary treatments. I went to the Bio Med Center in Providence, Rhode Island for five days of treatments. These were all using advanced technology and were very enjoyable, and I guess they were effective. I had what I had come to expect; "a healing crisis" came right afterwards. But I had no idea I would be covered with a red rash that was extremely uncomfortable for two months! I went to the internet and discovered that many others who had used too much cortisone were also suffering from "red rash syndrome". If I had kept up my membership with the National Eczema Association I would have known about this, but I hadn't.

❃　❦　❃　❦　❃

Most of the time that I was in an academic setting, I was not engaged with learning. There are many reasons for this, but once I started attending "workshops," I finally paid attention. Maybe this is because I am apparently a "right brain" person, and it was not until I experienced learning on an emotional level that I could feel interested enough to engage.

One image I like is seeing our lives as a needlework design. While we are alive, we see all the loose threads on the back of the design and cannot really make sense of it all. However, when we die, we see the masterpiece on the other side. We see the full picture of how it all worked out.

One thing I wish I had known when I was young is the importance of our choices. You may think this seems obvious, but it really is not, because our society and culture condition us and make us unaware of how they are shaping us. For example, we get the idea that we are supposed to be a certain way, and our individual tendency is just not given enough value.

Each of us is completely unique. We are often told this and that even every snowflake or grain of sand is different. But that insight never stuck; at least, it did not impress me until very recently. Frankly, this pandemic has for some reason enabled me to appreciate how phenomenally different we all are. I like that somehow I now understand that curiosity drives us toward certain areas of interest, and that is unique and telling.

I'll give you an example. Today I was on a Zoom call with two friends who live in NYC. I told them I had so enjoyed listening to Dani Shapiro reading her book *Inheritance* on Audible. They said they were in a book group and that they and all the others in the group did not like the book at all. They found it pretentious and some other negative judgment. Well, then I was able to see that one reason I was so spellbound by this book is that it discusses artificial insemination, and one of my sisters has children because of that procedure. No wonder I am fascinated by the story of a fifty-four-year-old woman suddenly discovering that the man she thought was her father actually was not. Her difficulty in finding her biological father and all that it entailed, I found enthralling. There are always reasons, I think, that we are grabbed by particular stories.

The point I want to make is related to this: each of us human beings has a very different experience on this planet. What is of interest for me is to connect and share my perspective. My particular life is one that has been shaped by my parents' separation the day I was born and by my lifetime struggle with eczema and learning disabilities. It was also very much affected by having three older brothers and four younger half siblings.

Our experiences are expressed in artistic endeavors, and it is satisfying to feel we have been seen and heard. I love writing class because I meet other brave Souls who share their lives through their writing. It is enormously satisfying to connect with others and see that, although each of us is unique, we often can identify with what others have lived through.

❋ ❦ ❋ ❦ ❋

I am hopeless at opening containers. Even little plastic ones with organic nuts in them. I pull back that transparent tab okay, but then lifting the lid is practically impossible. One of the many blessings of having dear Monica living with me is she is adept at opening all kinds of things. This is primarily because she has the patience I often lack.

She is also solid in her confidence, as far as I can see. She knows how to do stuff. I have stupidly allowed a broken picture frame to sit outside on my porch. In it is a photo of a lion. The large, framed photo was a gift from a neighbor when I lived in Lincoln. We had gone on a trip to South Africa together and were visitors at the famous game park, where we loved seeing lions. This is something I have always liked because I have a special fondness for lions, but to leave it to greet our mail carrier each day was really silly. She never commented on it. Why I put it there I am not really sure.

But yesterday I realized I had left it out there on my front porch for well over a week, clearly now with the glass broken. Then I brought it in last evening and put it on the dining room table, allowing me time to consider how to dispose of it. Do I attempt to keep the photo? The man who gave it to me has died after a long siege with Alzheimer's. The photo is faded and not really that good a photo, the frame is worthless, and the glass is just a worry. I consulted with Monica, and she carefully put the entire frame with photo and broken glass into a paper bag. She then carefully placed strips of tape over the top of the bag so that no one will get injured. The bag will be picked up on Tuesday without, we hope, anyone being hurt by the broken glass.

How is it that Monica is so capable, and yet I feel so helpless in anything that is mechanical? I have a small walker that my granddaughter used to use to get around my house. She has moved so I want to donate it to someone who can use it, but first I want to see if it can be made to help a friend who fell last week and needs one. I had to ask for help to see if moving various parts could make it be of any use. Was all my ineptitude due to a life of privilege? Certainly not; I know that not the case. But the impact of so much being done for me all these decades does leave a layer of guilt that I feel often.

Yes, the wealthy are unaware of a lot of their privileges. I had a very limited understanding of how my life compared to others, except from the contrast with friends at my private girls' school in NYC. In her book titled *You're Likely Not a Racist: Answers for Curious White People*, Teresa Reed tells us that we all have bias from the way we were raised. We are all blind in some sense, and we cannot know what we have not been taught. When I visited my mother in Beverly Farms, MA, I saw only the girls in my "outing class" (day camp), each of whom was as white and used to comforts as I was. One of them said the other day that when she was looking at her bank statement she was surprised to see a three-million-dollar deposit. It took her a few minutes, she told me, to realize that it was from the sale of her NYC apartment. She added, "This is great because now I can put it toward the cost of decorating my new apartment that is still being built on the West Side." Living in Rhinebeck, I have become good friends with women of very different backgrounds, and those same friends don't use Audible because of the extra cost per month.

※　❋　※　❋　※

Last night Monica mentioned that she would like to get some trays for her mother. "How about just taking two of mine?" I asked, having picked two with good edges and matching roosters in different colors.

"Oh, you don't mind?" Monica replied.

"You know, Monica, that I can't use all of these trays. I'd be delighted to give them to your mother," I reassured.

This morning Monica told me that she showed her mother the trays last night and that her mother wants to thank me for them. We are collecting a lot of things for Monica to send to St. Lucia for her family down there. She will pack all the china, glass, clothes, and so much more into big barrels. I am embarrassed by having a basement full of things that are not being used, and at least this will help some. I know that having less for my children to have to deal with is a help to them when that day comes. (As of this writing, I have decided to join a retirement community in Louisville, Kentucky, near two of my children and five grandchildren. This is a three-year plan and gives me a sense of security in this time of uncertainty.)

Yes, it is embarrassing to have so much, but I just do the best I can to respond when I can. I accept that the injustices are huge, but I am at least a bit more aware of them than I was when I was growing up!

❋ ❦ ❋ ❦ ❋

My daughter was nineteen months old, and I was living in NYC when my first son was born. We lived across from Lenox Hill Hospital, so I only had to cross the street to have a natural childbirth and was very excited. I had been reading about it since before my daughter was born, but because she had arrived "sunny-side up," my doctor said I definitely needed anesthesia so he could turn her around. I remember waking up in that recovery room asking the nurse whether I had had a boy or a girl.

This time, in October of 1970, I was determined not to be knocked out but to experience the birth naturally. I got into the elevator and then had another contraction. That passed, and the elevator man was relieved to see me walk across the street, hanging on to my husband's arm. I was relieved to have a wheelchair given to me as I walked into the side entrance of the hospital and was wheeled to the elevator so the nurse could take me up to the floor where my doctor was waiting. I said goodbye to my husband at that point.

The most vivid memory is of the nurse telling me fairly harshly to "PUSH!" I pushed with all my might but clearly was not succeeding. Finally, the nurse leaned on my belly and pushed hard as well. That is when I had a vision. I saw an enormous circle with people, animals, and all living things inside. Each had a light, and the light was love. I understood then that all of us are connected. Animals, plants, humans, the oceans ... all are part of the same source: love.

I remember that when my husband visited, I told him about my vision, and he said it was just the medications they had given me. I reminded him, "But I didn't have any medication. I had natural childbirth."

"Well, it is just some synapses doing something in your brain. It doesn't mean anything at all," he said confidently.

Years later, I was reading a book that described a mystical experience. That was when I realized I actually had one that day giving birth to my son. Then this morning, as I was reading my usual daily messages, Richard Rohr talked about "The Great Chain of Being." Rohr is a Catholic priest who wrote the following:

I would like to reclaim an ancient, evolving, and very Franciscan metaphor: the Great Chain of Being. This image helps us rightly name the nature of the universe, God, and the self, and to direct our future thinking. Scholastic theologians tried to communicate a linked and coherent world through this image. The essential and unbreakable links in the chain include the Divine Creator, the angelic heaven, the human, the animal, the world of vegetation, all water, and planet Earth itself with its minerals. In themselves, and in their union together, they proclaim the glory of God … and the inherent dignity of all things. This became the basis for calling anything and everything sacred.[5]

Now here I am this morning wondering how many of us have had experiences that we have not honored because of someone else's reaction to our experience.

As Brené Brown says, "Anger is a catalyst. Holding onto it will make us exhausted and sick […] It's an emotion that we need to transform into something life giving; courage, love, change, compassion, justice."[6] When I think about injustice to others and the anger that it creates, I wonder how we might transform that to make change.

---

5. Richard Rohr, *The Wisdom Pattern: Order, Disorder, Reorder* (Cincinnati: Franciscan Media, 2001), 148–149.

6. Brené Brown, *Atlas of The Heart: Mapping Meaningful Connection and the Language of Human Experience* (New York: Random House, 2021), 218.

The Hunting Ground, a documentary about college sexual assault, tells us that one out of four girls is sexually assaulted each year in college. This is in this, our United States. Can we use our outrage to work for change?

❋ ❦ ❋ ❦ ❋

It is February 3, 2020, and I am aghast at all that has happened in this year to shift my inner life. It began, of course, with Monica moving in the August before the 2019 pandemic. I immediately felt comforted by her company. In those first few months I did try to get her to like movies, but that was not going to happen.

This morning I am polishing the little saltshakers and shovels I found when Monica and I went through all my silver last week. They have sat on the counter near my toaster oven for days, and clearly Monica is not wanting to pull up the silver polish, so now I am doing that. Another little pleasure I get is emptying the dishwasher for her each morning. I have discovered that this little task takes just the amount of time that it takes my electric kettle to come to a boil for my tea, so it is a small gesture of gratitude that I enjoy.

When we went through the silver, I found a set of stainless steel that no one has used and is a hodge-podge of silverware that Monica says could be used in St. Lucia. So, she is deciding which of my unused items from the basement and elsewhere she can collect for the barrel that she will be sending "home" in March. Before that, she will be driven down to Brooklyn, where she has a room and retreats about once a month.

I feel so happy about the process of clearing out my basement. I have a friend come on Thursdays who helps me put some of the unclaimed china into boxes for my ten grandchildren, and yesterday Monica cleared up the basement, or at least organized it in a very tidy and helpful manner. I am no longer embarrassed by the mess that I have somehow allowed myself to accrue. This is an example of her assistance. She knows me as well as anyone, and my warts are visible and accepted, as it were.

❊　❦　❊　❦　❊

In January 2019, my friend Jessica and I flew to Georgia to spend a workshop with a medium named Suzanne. When I flew home, I had only one day before I went down to NYC to stay at the Cosmopolitan Club for a week to attend the program "Fearless Communicators." On that particular day, I was lying on my day bed in my downstairs bedroom when I remembered that Suzanne has a radio show, so I decided to tune in. It was a Thursday afternoon at 4:00 p.m. Of course, being tech challenged, I had difficulty and was prompted by the computer to just call in on my cell phone, which I succeeded in doing. I listened for about ten minutes and then got a call from my neighbor across the street.

I thought it was okay to pick up and chat with her, leaving the radio connection paused. After we chatted for five minutes, I was reconnected to the radio station and immediately heard Suzanne say, "Now I will answer questions randomly from you, but I do select ones that may not be waiting on hold. Alexandra, are you there? What is your question today?"

I was so thunderstruck that I could barely speak, but I managed to say, "I just returned from my weekend workshop with you in Savannah, and I guess I wish it had been for a month because I am finding it very difficult to believe in Spirit Guides." She responded by telling me to keep asking for help from my Guides and believing that they are helping me. It was such synchronicity, and I am glad that I can relisten to the recording of that astonishing call.

That next week in NYC, I was able to focus on the "Fearless Communicators" program. There were five young women in the group led by two amazing facilitators. I was given the honor of being called the "Elder" of the group and was asked to begin and end each of our sessions. This tribute alone had an astounding impact. I was looked at with respect, and it gave me a boost of confidence that lasted!

Getting up in front of about fifty strangers was not that hard for me, and I enjoyed their response. It built up, even as it was taking place, a feeling of confidence I have rarely experienced. I was able to respond to comments and be spontaneous, which is a characteristic I now cherish.

That evening, February 12, 2020, was life changing. Even as it was happening, I knew that my sense of Self was being transformed. Now I understand that just telling our stories enables healing to happen.

In fact, just three weeks ago my friend Sandy was over, and I was attempting to show her Dr. Zach Bush's four-minute workout but could not get the volume to work on my computer. In frustration, I looked up at the ceiling and said, "Guides, I need this volume to work," and, you guessed it, the volume immediately came on.

"Well, I sure am a believer now," Sandy laughed. It was a delightful moment of joy for us both.

Now, that reliance on my own judgment has been transferred to the pendulum. I was introduced to my first pendulum twenty years ago. It was pink and was a gift from a friend when we visited Switzerland together. I had put it away and forgotten about it, until summer before last when I came across it in my jewelry box. I was on a walk with my friend Kathy and wanted to tell her about it, but I could not remember the word "pendulum." At that exact moment, I looked to my left, and there in a shop window was a display of them with a sign saying "Pendulums"! We went into the shop, and I bought a turquoise one, which I handed to my grandson last week when he was here.

The enjoyment that I now get from using my pendulum to make decisions is both hilarious and fun. When I get the urge to write to someone, I ask my pendulum whether it is a good idea. I get an answer—frequently one that surprises me—and have no hesitation about following it. Why? Part of the fun is it is new and I trust it. With it being a time when we don't know what to believe, especially with so much censorship going on, I am amused and delighted by depending on this particular object.

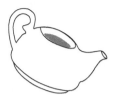

CHAPTER 9

Finding Compassion
for Myself

*Ask yourself: Is there joy, ease, and lightness
in what I am doing? If there isn't, then time
is covering up the present moment and life
is perceived as a burden or a struggle.*

—Eckhart Tolle

I have a bruised coccyx. I went for a walk in the lovely orchard where my friend lives, lost my footing, and just happened to fall on mostly grass, but my tail bone hit a wedge of rock. I was amazed by how much it hurt right away and thought I might have done some serious damage, but I had not.

I even managed to get up after my fall, albeit not easily. By then my friend noticed I was not where she was and came back to find me. I told her I was fine and immediately said, "This will be a reminder of my need to walk exceedingly gingerly. My balance is lousy, and I need to pay attention."

I never knew that not feeling self-conscious was a goal of mine. But it is. I wish to feel sufficiently confident in who I am to no longer worry about appearances.

What does it mean to be comfortable with oneself? And if I truly am, will I be able to actually say how I feel?

✳   ❋   ✳   ❋   ✳

This week I made a few mistakes. What pleases me is that my apology for being impulsive was accepted! I no longer beat myself up for hours about making a mistake, and this is progress.

This afternoon I wish to rewrite a toast to my son, who is soon to celebrate his fiftieth birthday. I wrote one and then had a friend film me speaking it so that I can do what my daughter-in-law requested: put the video into a drop box that will then be edited and sent to my son on his birthday, along with who knows how many others.

What I feel I should do is think of particular things and say them with humor and then memorize my toast so

I can sound off-the-cuff but actually be well-prepared. The extent of my (and my friends of similar age) discomfort with technology is probably not appreciated by the younger generations.

In April, my niece wrote me an email requesting a two-minute video of me wishing my sister a very happy birthday. I worked at what I hoped would be both genuine and perky for her. When I told my daughter how I was struggling to do it, my daughter even reminded me, "You did a good job on that Fearless Communicators video, Mom. Why is this such a big deal?"

With this in mind, I walked out the front door to the back yard, got myself situated near my trampoline, pushed the video button, proceeded to give a two-minute speech for my sister, and pressed the button again. What I did not know until after the actual birthday was that all that came through was the top of my head with no sound. Apparently I had pushed the video button as I went out the front door, and all anyone could see was the top of my head and my walking somewhere. The time that I thought I had turned it on, I actually turned it off! There was no audio at all.

I cannot think of a time when I brought such good cheer to my four children. They laughed so hard they had tears. Each brought their children in to watch their Nonnie trying to make a video, which brought quite a bit of humor, even if unintended. But my main point is that I don't want to have to memorize my toast to my son. I can read it and not have it be obvious that I am reading it, but it needs to have specifics in it.

Until recently, I did not know how much I like to plan. Last night I met a woman at Omega who told me she had recently sold her house near mine here in the village of Rhinebeck. She said, "I love Omega and I love to plan, so when I saw land for sale, I grabbed it." She explained that she had built a house and is so happy. I told her I love to plan as well, and now I realize why this next example has come about.

When my youngest child came to visit with his three little ones—ages seven, six, and four—I loved having them for the few days they were here. But it made me think about how I have a huge basement full of toys that they enjoy for only for only a short time each year. I then began thinking of all the maintenance costs I am paying, plus the size of this wonderful house, and I impulsively called a real estate broker friend to ask her to come over.

That friend told me she would put a low number on the house and create a bidding war if I decided to put it on the market and that I certainly would never have any trouble selling this house. It only took me one day to realize how much I love living here and I decided to keep the house, at least for now. Then I calculated how my three grandchildren who now store things in my basement would be out in four years. By then they will have graduated from college, and unless the younger one chooses a college near me, my identity as "the grandmother with the comfy place to stay" might shift.

When I discussed the idea of my perhaps moving into a full-care facility in a few years, Monica was completely supportive. She told me she would love to possibly move home to St. Lucia when I decide to move, which confirmed my decision to get on the list for a place. It makes me happy to take control of something! That is why I want to do this. I can focus on positive change and make sure that I clear out my house myself and recycle my belongings to people I care about. Otherwise, I feel as if I am just waiting to die here. I like change, and I especially like being able to choose a new environment. So, I am pleased to have made a momentous decision with ease. Of course, I may change my mind, and I like that too.

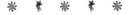

Today I am working on my aspiration board. As my homework for tonight's support group meeting, I will draw some words in different colors on a piece of paper. I realize there are only two more sessions before this group is over, and I want to create some aspirations before our next Zoom meeting.

My aspirations include regular meditation, listening to more music, and reading at a particular time each day. This is because I realize how much I like structure in this odd time we are living through, and if I don't make these aspirations a part of my daily life, the time slips away. Yes, I do enjoy talking with my friends on the phone, but no longer will I sacrifice my reading time by talking it all away.

The first word for my board, as it is one quality I would like to learn, is patience. Monica has demonstrated this for me over and over again, and I am learning more about what patience means.

Another aspiration is to work hard. I confess that over the decades some habits are especially hard to break. One of them is "winging it." It is something like multitasking, a skill that I got good at doing. Now is the time to unlearn those two skills, because I wish to slow down and actually work at a task.

The last aspiration I want on this board is to write. I have been doing more of it since I began my writing group, and for that I am profoundly grateful. I listened to David Sedaris on Master Class and really was inspired to write daily. I do enjoy it.

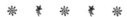

Last night I had my two teenage granddaughters and their mother over for supper on my porch. My daughter and I consumed two bottles of wine and had a fairly good time. But I noticed that I was staring at each of these long-blond-haired beauties of sixteen and eighteen with intensity.

I wondered why they left rather quickly when I went inside for something. They each carried stuff in and graciously said goodbye, but there was an abruptness to their 2:00 a.m. departure that I decided was due to my referencing myself too much.

I realize that I probably do this because these girls are here for only two more months. Their mother, my older daughter, is moving out of Rhinebeck to Louisville, KY, where her brother lives with his family. I am totally thrilled that they will all be together, and my daughter needs to start a new chapter because her divorce is now final. I get it, but it means I will not often have their full attention. Somehow, I have been trying to cram everything I have come to believe into whatever small spaces of time I get with them. I now think this is because I am getting old and realize I must let go, but doing so is damn tough.

My other daughter is also leaving Rhinebeck, and that means her two children will also soon be in LA and far away from their Nonnie. I am realizing that the desire to hold on to them is not something I can do, so I will try to let all four grandchildren go and wish my two daughters farewell in as good a manner as I can.

What I see now is that my self-centered conversations are really just ways for me to try to pass on my "wisdom," and doing so is useless! This realization is a pin prick to my ego, but when I look through a spiritual lens, this is a good thing because it is lessening my ego's strength. I think this means I am unconsciously preparing for my own death!

What is new for me is that I actually feel compassion for myself today, and for that I am grateful.

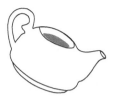

CHAPTER 10

Embracing Uncertainty

*A letter is in fact the only device for combining
solitude and good company.*

—Jacques Barzun

Sometimes we forget that a lot of progress has been made in our society. In my youth, many children who were brought up with upper-class English heritage were given very little physical affection. The expectation in Victorian times was for children to behave well, but there was not a lot of hugging or encouragement. When I was a teenager, I saw families ashamed of having anyone suffering with a mental illness, and it was appalling for anyone to have a child out of wedlock. It was beyond terrible if a young person fell in love with someone of a different background or, God forbid, a different skin color! So, some strides have been made.

The other night, President Joe Biden was trying to say that there has actually been a lot of progress in civil rights but that those stories of progress have not been told with much emphasis. I will only say that I think more has improved than we realize at this moment. We have to keep believing that or we might give up the struggle.

How hard it is for me to know how to handle my own outrage and anger. I am here in complete comfort and relative safety and still feel fairly helpless. Today has been especially weird. One daughter and grand-daughter were here on the front porch for a long time, and another granddaughter came and joined them there as I was having peppermint tea with yet another grand-daughter in the living room. Earlier I was outside with two of them while my grandson was out with a friend playing on their bikes. A neighbor came by and sat with us, but none of us were having much fun. It was so strange and sad.

I said something like, "I am mourning" when my granddaughter asked how I was. She said she was, too, but it did not add up to any good conversation. Then a friend from NYC called, and I realized from our phone conversation that she and her partner have been having a really hard time due to losing their jobs. The amount of suffering is truly impossible to process. I wish I knew something that could help.

At least tomorrow Monica and I are going over to help a neighbor clean her pool house, which I am truly looking forward to. It will be a satisfying and helpful way to thank her for her generosity with her pool.

But right now, for the first time since this pandemic began, I am helping myself to a glass of wine. Monica is cooking a shepherd's pie and I am sitting in the dining room typing this while I await my dinner. Why the wine? I feel sort of spacey and need to understand that I can ask for some help from my Spirit Guides. I am asking for that now because I want to be able to write something that will help someone. I am reminded of the book by Annie Grace called *The Alcohol Experiment*. This is a thirty-day challenge to interrupt habits and take control of one's drinking. It has helped several people close to me, and because of my mother's alcoholism I am eager to share ways of helping heal addictions.

My friends help heal me too. This morning, for example, a dear friend came by. We sat for a while out on my back porch and enjoyed some time, but I stupidly answered a phone call from another friend. I must learn not to do that! The friend told me that I am someone with hope and therefore am peaceful to be around. I feel so far from that right now and need to grasp that compliment from earlier today and hold on to it.

If I can trust in God, then I may be able to put the world's suffering into a new place in my mind. The lens of faith is one I am striving to look through. I want to hope that this national expression of outrage will bring about positive change. There are young leaders out there, and I am praying for them to have the courage and clarity to help us create a new society. If they can be led to how best to act right now, I will rejoice.

I know there are organizations that are focusing their efforts on supporting leaders in knowing how best to take action for social justice. Somehow, however, when I see emails from some of these organizations, I don't bother to read them. This is shameful, and I will now go and look at them because to not do so is wrong. If I truly want to do something, and they are an organization that I have supported for decades, I can at least read what they are saying.

What is it that makes me hesitate? Why have I not already sent a check to the food project my friend is involved in? Why do I ignore emails? What exactly are my values? I feel as though my privileged life is now showing in neon signs, and I feel ashamed by how little I do and how paralyzed I feel.

❋　❦　❋　❦　❋

I have often thought if I were to live this life again, or reincarnate, I would like to be a wet nurse. That way my breastfeeding would benefit a baby, and I would feel the satisfaction that I felt when I was doing that for my children.

This tells me of my need to feel satisfied that my giving is sufficient. I recall with such delight the babies all being so glad to be satisfied, full, and drifting off to sleep. When my daughters were here today, I was conscious of their trying to spend time with me before they leave, but their time with one another was far more satisfying than their time with me. That is natural, and when I can accept that I will be more content. I am trying to live in the moment, savor them, and let them go. It helps to listen to podcasts that soothingly say how best to allow this transformation in outlook occur. I particularly like listening to Tara Brach.

I have written about disappointment and realize mine is so minor compared to others' that I am ashamed for even talking about it. But in my effort to be honest about what a distressing period of time this is, I am including it.

❋　❋　❋　❋　❋

In August of 2020, after both of my daughters had left Rhinebeck, I went to Winifred's little red house on Oak Road and began learning about this ancient Chinese

way of healing called Qigong. I was greeted with a mug
of delicious tea sweetened with honey.

After a little introduction, I was clear about the
importance of what would become my daily twenty-
minute practice of exercises that Master Lu has developed. The Dragon's Way is an exercise I have been able
to do daily for six months now.

That first day with my tea, Winifred explained that
the only way I could benefit was by being really faithful
about this practice. When I saw that the exercises were
not especially difficult or even enormously strenuous,
I was encouraged. That was when I made the commitment to myself to keep this up. I like to experiment with
almost anything that promotes healing, so I signed on.

After I finished my tea, I climbed up on Winifred's
massage table and put myself in her experienced hands.
Frankly, I have no idea what her hands do because
after a very enjoyable few minutes of massage, I fall
fast asleep. One time it took three attempts to wake me
before she could get me to stir from wherever it was
I went!

This Friday, Winifred is arriving at my house at
8:00 a.m. to interview me about the results of this practice. I have been thinking about this so I will be ready
to tell her. The most obvious result at the moment is my
huge increase in appetite. Yesterday I defrosted a strip
steak to eat, half for lunch and the other half for dinner.
But when I smelled it cooking, I realized I wanted all

of it for lunch. I wolfed it down with two large baked potatoes and some broccoli. That afternoon I put in an entire chicken to roast and devoured almost all of it for an early dinner at six. When I mentioned this over the phone to Winifred, she said this is very common. She, too, becomes ravenous periodically. "It is all part of the process, Alexandra," she told me. "Your body is functioning well, and this is all part of the healing."

Most remarkable to me is the way my eczema has cleared up so that I only have a little on the palms of my hands. All the places that used to be red and itchy have disappeared, and with that I am able to be more relaxed and less anxious. My concentration is better, and I am better able to prioritize.

My relationship to my children has also shifted. I can step back more easily and realize that they are launched, and I can focus now on my own life. This is good because I am writing now, which is flowing more easily.

Exactly what Winifred does I really don't know. What I do know is that I have benefited enormously from my weekly sessions with her.

❋ ❋ ❋ ❋ ❋

Just a few minutes before writing class this morning, I noticed a squirrel eating on a small wrought-iron table next to an old-fashioned lamp out on my back porch.

I got out my phone and snapped three photos of this gray creature. I did take note of this rather odd behavior because, honestly, I dislike squirrels. But this time of sequestering in place has led me to be aware, more than I used to be, of all life.

Another example of this happened yesterday when I saw a small spider in my upstairs bathroom. I hesitated quite a few minutes before talking myself into grabbing a tissue, picking up the live creature, squishing it, and placing it in the toilet before flushing it away from my thoughts and space. Years ago, I attended several Buddhist retreats. In one of them, there was a vow to not kill any living thing. I have to admit that broken vow has haunted me on a regular basis for decades now. I am so horrendously full of contradictions, most of which are too revealing to give to you this morning, but this tiny admission to just a smidgin of guilt over killing a weeny little spider will suffice for now.

Actually, what this leads me to is the importance of the decisions we make. I am fascinated by the importance of what we do commit to. I was so pleased with myself when I realized I had chosen to not be bitter after my divorce from my first husband. That may be when I began examining my decision-making with some care.

❋　❋　❋　❋　❋

This morning I got a call from a friend of mine who lives in a facility in Massachusetts for those who need a fair amount of care. She has spent most of her life in psychiatric facilities and has just returned from a two-month stay in one near the assisted living place where she now resides. Sadly, she is quarantining because she had to go to the emergency room three times and each of those requires more quarantining. She has little ability to deal with technology, and when I ask if there is someone to help, she always says, "not really." Our conversations are awkward for me, but I have kept our connection. She texts me each Sunday. She never fails unless she is in the hospital

Yesterday she told me that the worst part of being in the hospital is that they kept her on a very restricted diet due to her diabetes being way out of control. "I was always hungry, Alexandra," she would say, "and so I would hide my food. I put a banana in my bedside drawer, and no one caught me." She laughed but then went on to say that she got even more secretive and hid food under her mattress.

This reminded me of another family member who was recently in a psychiatric hospital as well. After finding food she had been hiding under her mattress and witnessing her screaming and shouting at the person who was trying to help her, her caretaker called for an ambulance. When two men tried to get her onto the gurney to put her in the ambulance, she ranted and threw a glass that shattered everywhere. Her eighteen-year-old son witnessed the whole thing, and I cannot imagine how horrifying that must have been.

Trying to maneuver my attention in a positive direction each day takes all of my energy. I want to believe in Spirit Guides, and I do (most of the time). That way I can request guidance about which foot to put in front of the other foot and trust that what I wish to do is adequate. Knowing there is so much suffering, in so many ways, can take a toll. The pandemic is just another level of suffering added to the separation, fear, and inequality that has already been going on.

When we are told to be patient and just see what comes forth, it certainly is a surprise. I am not sure what I hoped for, but I remember starting out thinking I would write about how my soul was not prepared for this life I have lived. That is a strange admission. I think I became hardened at various times in my life, but then I was clearly broken many times. Perhaps it is that process that has actually softened me. I am now able to live with, if not embrace, uncertainty.

I like to think I am now resting in a curious certainty; that is, nothing is ever wasted in our lives. I am able to trust that life will shape me, and perhaps it is this trust that makes me say I have never felt as content as I do these days. I have a routine and it is working for me. Monica and I get on so well and she seems deeply content. I believe that her influence, just her very being, is what has enabled me to quiet down and take in her calm demeanor. No one would call me calm, even now, but most of my friends and maybe even my children sense a positive change.

I wonder how these two women struggling with lifelong psychiatric conditions would react if they were to hear these thoughts?

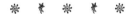

What is the etiquette these days about how grandparents should be treated? When I was a child, my mother felt she had to visit her mother every day! We lived only a five-minute drive away from my grandmother Gaga's house, but it was what we called a "command performance" I was well aware that neither my grandmother nor my mother enjoyed the ten minutes we spent together, so I was bewildered as to why it was necessary.

When my children were teenagers, I told them I did not want to have them be burdened by manners that were not real. I did not insist on showing respect for one's elders, though, and I kind of regret that now. Trying to let go of children and grandchildren is especially relevant for me now because both of my daughters who live here in Rhinebeck have put their houses on the market and will be moving within two months.

I don't think either of them will have any problem selling their homes, so I have a reason to rejoice. But having them move away is sad for me, and I am realizing how important it is for me to let them go. I am enthusiastic for each of my daughters to start new chapters and only hope I can stay in relatively close touch.

This is the sticky part. How close in proximity do we all want to be? How do we figure this out? I listened today to Reese Witherspoon and Kerry Washington being interviewed by Brené Brown about their acting in *Little Fires Everywhere*. This mini-series is all about mothering and it is exceedingly well done. Witherspoon's character seems to have it all together, and I related to this character and the mask of perfection. Washington's character, on the other hand, seems to be unraveled. It is not until the end that we see all of us are imperfect parents. However, the topic of raising children has always been of enormous interest to me. In fact, I would rather discuss this than go to a concert, visit a museum, or go on a cruise.

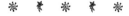

As I think you know, my generation was brought up to be certain we hand wrote thank-you notes to those who had sent us gifts at Christmas and birthdays. There is a photo of me at age ten on Christmas afternoon knocking them off while we were visiting the Groton Plantation.

I always finished my thank-you notes on Christmas Day. Even when I was on my honeymoon in 1966, I finished all the notes to thank the many people who had sent us gifts. I don't think it occurred to either of us to question why I was the only one doing the thanking, but I recall feeling very accomplished when I checked off all the names and put the last stamp on that final envelope.

Nowadays, my friends and I compare notes about the responses or lack thereof that we receive from grandchildren. We no longer require handwritten notes, but we do expect at least a text or, even better, a phone call to acknowledge our efforts. We very seldom get either.

What I have noticed is that my pleasure in finding a book for each of the grandkids at Christmas is definitely heightened by slipping a fifty-dollar bill into each book before wrapping it. Each year I hope to get a phone call to say how they feel about the book that I have chosen, but I am often disappointed.

I know they don't mean to be rude, but I have hoped that they at least understand I want a connection with each of them. It is not "pro forma" that they must send a note but rather that they make an effort in acknowledging I have gone lengths to please them. But more importantly, the hope is that the gift and thank you exchange creates a reason for us to talk with one another.

This is what I feel has been lost in this change in family norms. We are left feeling not only unappreciated but also unacknowledged. Can they see this? Do they care? I wonder if I would be able to discuss this topic with them without our becoming defensive. What my job is now is to redo my expectations by recognizing that a new culture is forming and letting go of old rules that no longer apply. Most of my grandchildren's generation feel they don't need to respond to texts, and I am learning to no longer take it personally.

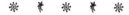

One of the conversations that I ruminate about is one I had with my elder daughter about a year ago. I had just finished reading *Dying to be Me* by Anita Moorjani and was on fire about this memoir about Moorjani's near-death experience. She had terminal cancer and tells her story on Audible, my favorite way to hear stories. She died and went to such a loving space that she did not want to return. But she talked with her father, who had died years earlier, and he told her it was not her time and that she needed to help people live and stop being so frightened of dying. Her return-from-death story moved me.

I told my daughter and many close friends about Moorjani's story. I had already read other books about near-death experiences and knew the phenomenon was explained away by those who are unaware of an invisible world, but I was already a believer. The story was pivotal in erasing my fear of death, or so I told my friends.

When I finished informing my daughter of this extraordinary account, I said how much I hoped she would read it. She paused and then sort of slowly said, "Mom, do you not remember that you told me about this book when it was first out, about five years ago?"

I was stunned, hurt, bewildered, and a bit angry. I want so much to be able to write about what it feels like to lose my memory, a particularly searing quality. I hope I can convey why I was so undone by this news: I don't care a hoot about forgetting people's names or even specific events or trips I have taken, but this was an inner shift that I thought was brand new. In fact, not only was the shift not new, but my reading of the book in 2019 that I told my friends was life changing had not had the impact I had bragged about. I wonder how many of them I had previously told that my life was utterly changed. Had I told them that same exact proclamation five years ago?

Now my goal is to start over again and again. Each day gives me a new opportunity to pay attention. Yes, I want to be able to listen and be aware of what is happening in a particular moment. One reason I like the classes I take now so much is that they give me practice at paying attention. Often the reason I forget things is because I am on autopilot and not attending to a specific action.

I blame a lot of my "memory loss" on not being in the present. But was that what happened after reading Moorjani's book five years ago? I am wondering why it did not stick, and I am fed up with that kind of rumination. Why ask those questions now? Maybe all I can focus on at this moment is what my intention is each day.

One of my main themes for 2021 is to accept what is. Surely, implied in this focus is my learning to forgive myself and move on to what is happening today, right now.

When interviewed by Oprah Winfrey, Goldie Hawn once shared that when she was eleven, she was asked what she wanted to be. She had been told that perhaps she would like to be a dancer or an actress, but her intention was clear, she said, and has always been consistent: "I want to be happy."[7]

---

7. "Golden Girl: Goldie Hawn on Happiness," Oprah.com, January 26, 2011, https://www.oprah.com/oprahshow/goldie-hawn-on-happiness/all.

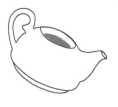

CHAPTER 11

Trusting Myself

*Giving voice to what is inner is essential
to surviving what is outer. No matter where
we live or whom we love, no matter what we
want or what we can't have.*

—Mark Nepo

W hile I have been on this healing path for quite some time, most recently I can see the incessant search for peace within and have learned that it is an inner/outer thing. We have to work on our healthy self-care to heal our wounds so that we can bring healing to our planet. No time is more important than right now with this global pandemic, which has caused me to go *in* more than ever before.

I have been reading about trauma, primarily by Gabor Maté and Bessel van der Kolk. While it is hard for me to really stay with all they are saying, I am mesmerized, and it has put me on a path to understanding what these two have discovered. My intention is to open people up to what these doctors and authors have proven.

I am hoping to help my grandchildren see these Healing Circles—mental, spiritual, and physical—and all the ways to understand ourselves in order to heal. In the Healing Circles I facilitate, everyone sits in a circle. It reminds me of the vision I saw when Michael was born, when all of life was represented in a circle, and the whole point is love.

We are all connected.

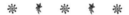

I have been asked to lead a new members group on Zoom for the local office of the "Rhinebeck at Home" organization. Currently, schools are still closed, masks (double ones) are recommended, and social distancing is being demanded by our government.

Who asked my generation how we would feel about lockdown and the sacrifices that others are making on our behalf, since we are considered the most vulnerable? At seventy-seven years old, I wish I was last in line for the vaccine rather than being pushed to the front.

For someone like me, a privileged person, I could probably have a compassionate death. I am well-connected, so I would most likely be given a "comfort pack" from hospice, which includes medications that can relieve symptoms in terminally ill patients. I am fortunate in not being afraid of death, but like most everyone, I don't want to suffer. I just heard a palliative care nurse talk about the reality of running out of some of the medications that would relieve suffering patients because of COVID-related shortages. So, this is a major worry for us elders.

I am more than willing to leave this life I love if it means my grandchildren could go to school again. But I am trying to ask about the millions of people who are starving to death at this juncture in this pandemic. What are we doing about them?

I am frustrated by the enormously complex results of the decisions that have been made for us. Who debated the initial steps to close businesses and ruin millions of lives? I hear that little four- and five-year-olds are no longer holding hands when in line but are masked and told to hold their hands behind their backs! What will this do to this entire generation of children?

One question we need to examine is our relationship to risk. This is a very important query, but no one I know is debating it within my world, which is one of the problems. I have found the news somewhat unhelpful and inaccurate, and I now watch it hardly at all. I don't say a word about my misgivings when speaking with others, because I don't want to be looked upon as a listener to conspiracy theories. That is simply not the case.

I wish wise elders were being asked their opinions on media, but I hear none. There is some wisdom in the YouTube world, but somehow a lot of what is out there does not last long due to censorship. Of course, a lot of it may also be inaccurate. When I tell this to my son who is a law professor, I feel inept at explaining how I know this, but I have friends who have watched this happen.

I know what I believe, but for those who have been raised to trust the media it is inconceivable for many to question its "truth." But our beliefs don't hold up against facts that are presented by those we don't agree with. I am actually surprised by my own beliefs, but I know that this way of handling this health crisis is at least partially wrong. I have come to trust my own judgment as well as my intuition, at least more than I used to.

We need community. We have known this forever. That is how healing takes place. Stories are told, and this can bring about extraordinary transformation. At this time, all human beings are being ordered *not* to be together. Thank God for Zoom because at least we are telling our stories on that platform.

I know that I have an enviable life, and I am still feeling the effects of being cut off from my family and friends. What can I do? Try to live in the moment and do small gestures of kindness. I can share my vulnerability, and I think that is what I am doing here.

I am someone who loves to plan, and I have a new calendar about to arrive. I use four a year because it makes me happy to start a fresh one, neatly writing in pencil. By the time I order my new calendar, the old one looks appallingly messy with eraser marks and ink splatters and such. But the peace I feel when I begin the new calendar is palpable. I repeat those things that invariably bring me pleasure.

Since I have lived most of my life in the future, one thing I am learning is to try to be present—to be in the moment. One of my dear friends down the street from me has just started chemo. She had tumors removed from her spinal cord and was then told she has lung cancer. She endured a whole series of radiation treatments and is now having her husband bring her the eight daily pills that she downs with yogurt. I want to visit this friend, but they are in lockdown. I might be bringing the virus, so no one is welcome to sit next to her and hold her hand. Instead, I try to think of what she might like to read or what I can send her to eat.

Yesterday my friend Sandy called. She is eighty-three and fell over a cord in her house, but she did not break any bones. She is in a lot of pain from the fall, and when I suggested Epsom salts, she said she cannot get out of the bathtub on her own, so that rules out that potential source of comfort.

How do we nourish our hearts and Souls during this weird time? I have never been much of a poetry person, but during this time I find I like the soothing nature of poems. Meditation has also become something I like because it is comforting and predictable.

One surprise I am experiencing is that although I have always thought of myself as an extrovert and still I think I am, I am thoroughly appreciating all this time to reflect, read, write, and watch movies or other things I like on TV or the internet. I guess my introvert side is having a field day, having never been listened to before. We each have a story, and that is part of mine. Now I am hoping to use this time to integrate my many Selves. "Inner work" is not dull, and I am grateful for all the help I have been given from psychotherapy.

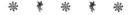

This past year has changed me more than any previous one. At least, this is what I think. Perhaps my first or second year of life actually was as profound, but I don't remember those and am happy to instead focus on this past year, 2020.

I can now go to sleep between 8:00 and 9:00 p.m. and get up between 3:00 and 5:00 a.m. every day. I have a routine that includes making myself a pot of English Breakfast tea, putting on the fire, turning on the lamp, then striking a match to light a large white candle that sits on an ottoman piled with books. I then read a Mary Oliver poem from *Devotions* and two other daily readings before I reach for my lovely journal. I write only a page, but I enjoy the process.

Time seems to go by very rapidly. I am astonished to see in my calendar that another weekend has arrived. Clearly something is altering my perception of time, and I only ascribe it to part of the mystery of the energies that are swirling about. I don't feel rushed and can go about my activities with less anxiety than I used to carry.

At the end of each and every day I do a meditation practice. I have never been able to focus like this before, but now the company of a few women on Zoom has become a comfort. It is like a warm comfy blanket that I climb under, wrapping up my day so I can relax into the evening.

What is a surprise to me is how little I miss going out to dinner with friends, traveling, and rushing around trying to get things done. There has been a major shift internally for me. No longer feeling the need to prove that I have a right to a space on our planet, I am more relaxed. I have rushed through all the decades and at last am feeling peaceful. This has increased both my gratitude and confidence. I write with more ease and enjoy writing in a new way.

The value that I put on friendship is not a change, but I savor my conversations with friends. One of my friends has fourth-stage cancer. We touch base nearly every day on FaceTime, and this is a blessing for us both. The reciprocity of friendship and its potential for mutual healing is a new awareness.

I am also much less compelled to keep up with my siblings. I always used to feel that I had to check in with them., but now I can trust that they will be taken care of without my attention. I remain responsive to them when they reach out but no longer feel responsible for them in the same way I used to.

I trust myself more and, most importantly, I have come to trust life. I realize now that my mind was not ready for much of what I have read or learned in the last fifty years. I am a "seeker." I have grabbed at workshops, books, and people. I now believe that my Soul led me to exactly the right people and healing modalities.

Because I am a woman of enormous privilege, I have had phenomenal opportunities. Often my mind, body, or Spirit could not take in what was offered, but I now see that the soil of my mind was not yet fertile. The seeds I planted are finally beginning to blossom.

❋ ❦ ❋ ❦ ❋

There is so much happening all over our globe, and I am aware of an infinitesimal piece of it, yet I know that I don't want to look away.

The prayer that I hold is for our human awareness to evolve and that we all become more conscious.

Just realizing that animals and plants are alive and that this connects us to them, isn't this progress? Can we change our behavior? Can we possibly recognize that love is what connects us? Can I look at everything with reverence? I pray to learn to do this.

On the other hand, there is the outcome of this dreadful lockdown situation. All those decisions made without our input, such as the closing of businesses and schools, have led to a horrifying rise in suicides, especially among teenagers, and deaths from starvation!

Now, whoever is in charge, and I don't know who they are, have control over the media. Resistance to the manipulation is shut down. We are being ordered to get vaccinated. We read that travel will be restricted to those who have been given one of these experimental drugs, but I don't want to take this shot because I believe I don't need it and that it is not safe.

The fear has spread so effectively that even my four intelligent, wonderful offspring believe we are all in desperate need of a vaccine. Just two days ago I was told that my younger son and his family would need to reconsider our trip in May to meet in Washington, DC, and my two children from Louisville, KY, would not welcome me to visit there unless I had the vaccine. I feel their protective love, but I loathe the fear.

This dilemma led me to pray in a very urgent way. Within a few minutes, my perspective shifted. I saw that my priority is my children and grandchildren, and that my opinions are mine to keep. I believe prayer handed me the key to my prison cell. I now can go ahead, get the shot, and still hold on to my opinions.

I think the chances of my getting COVID-19 are extremely slim. If I do get it, I will be able to treat it and recover, and if I don't, I will die sooner than I might have without it. But dying is no longer something I am frightened by. It is suffering that I wish to avoid, and considering my privileged life, I can get medications to ease that.

My friends and neighbors are racing to get their shots while there are many intelligent medical people saying it is not safe. I may be turned away because of having spent years on cortisone and having allergies, but I will show up for the vaccine at 11:45 a.m. next Monday, March 15th. My children are rejoicing, and my love for them drives me to do this.

❋　❋　❋　❋　❋

An Elder's Deep Love for Family

This Elder cherishes her children and grandchildren.
She believes she doesn't need the vaccine.
Death no longer frightens her.
What scares her is society's ability to instill fear and
division within families.
This is the virus we Elders want to eradicate.

Families naturally want to be together.
Grandparents want to be with their children and
grandchildren.
So, this Elder will get the experimental vaccine.
Her family is grateful that their Elder has chosen to be
with them this spring.
Can you feel the Elder love that is being showered on
you right now?

❋　❦　❋　❦　❋

I am eager for you to hear about where I believe my intuition has led me this past year. I am not someone who does research, but as soon as we were being told how important it was for businesses to close down, I got a strong sense of "Wait a minute. Where is the debate about this?"

When three friends of mine told me that there was some censorship going on, I listened and asked how they knew this. They told me they had found doctors speaking out about Dr. Fauci and how he was not the person to listen to. I was sent the link and was impressed by the video from California that included nurses and other doctors who were alarmed by the fast pace of the decisions. They pointed out the many medical problems that would be exacerbated by the focus on this virus, which they were saying still very little research had been done on it. When I went back to find the link to send to my son, it had been removed.

One of these friends who feels passionately against the media's way of telling us the news told me she had found many of the respected opponents being taken off social media. Why did I choose to listen to these three friends from different places? Each of them I respected, admired, trusted, and loved. I was also deeply pleased to have my intuition confirmed.

A week after my first shot of the Moderna vaccine, I was in the local hospital with severe vertigo, nausea, and extreme unsteadiness. A neurologist saw that my B12 was very low, so I had four weekly injections of that vitamin. The unsteadiness is still there, but it is not as severe as it was when I was in the emergency room. I had several nurses tell me that quite a few other people who had received the Moderna vaccine had come in with the same symptoms.

My thinking about the vaccine has caused my family and friends to look at me with some surprise. I am trying to gently disagree with those who are terrified of getting COVID-19, so I shift the conversations and make a note to keep listening to those who look at what is going on from a different perspective. I have become intrigued by those who channel from the spiritual realm. This is to explain that in the past year I am far more conscious of the existence of spirits. I think we each have a Soul and that this energy lives on after we die.

My four children were concerned about me because I insisted that I did not want to get the vaccine. Eventually they persuaded me to get it because otherwise I would not have been able to see them or my grandchildren. That is how strongly they were convinced by what they were being told in the mainstream media.

It is unusual for me to be so opposed to what my family and most of my friends believe. But I have felt so adamant that I wonder if it is a reflection of my Soul's intuition. I am learning to stay out of the political discussions, and I have never enjoyed those, so that is not so hard. But I am also determined to go on record for resisting the pressures that are being exerted on our society here in the United States. I am especially horrified by the "othering" of the unvaccinated!

It is essential for my well-being to be in as good a relationship with each of my grandchildren and children as possible, so now I keep quiet on this topic. But I am known for not accepting much of what we are told. For example, one of my friends has spoken with nurses in Australia who say that all the hospitals are filled with people who have been vaccinated, but the press tells us that it is the unvaccinated who are suffering in the hospitals. So, it is a big problem for each of us to determine for ourselves who to listen to and what to watch.

My younger son recently told me that he feels I do not need to get the booster shot. Interestingly, during a conversation with my other son about masks and school closings, he asked me, "Mom, are you willing to admit that you may be wrong?" I asked him the same. Of course, we admit that, but I have refused to get any of the booster shots.

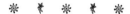

Dear Rumi,

Thank you for your poem "The Guest House." It has helped me during this last year. When I was unsettled, I would recall your message and examine my feelings. I could then sit with the discomfort and become introspective. I asked myself, "What am I learning from all this confusion?"

I have a friend named Jennifer who was furious with me for not being pro-mask. I will put one on when I am required to, but I have chosen to allow myself to not wear one when on my porch with visitors. I ask a guest if they would be more comfortable if I wear one, and if they say they would, then I comply.

But when Jennifer heard through the rumor mill that I was having lots of people over and we were not wearing masks, she stopped speaking to me. I thought of your words, and I realized when I went deeper in my thinking that I could be my own boss on my own front porch.

This has resulted in my becoming more confident. I realize that I need to consider my behavior and be courteous, but I can think for myself. We are all living through this time, and following your wise words can help us. I can accept Jennifer's anger, notice what it does to me, and acknowledge the hurt, but I can keep going on.

The other emotion that has come up repeatedly is deep sadness. When I am reminded of all the schools being closed and children being ordered to wear masks, I feel helpless and angry as well as sad. What can I learn from this? Anger and sadness have brought me clearer knowledge of who I am, what I can change, and what I cannot.

I have no control over school closings, but I can choose my own behavior. I can resist wearing a mask, at least on my own porch. This is a bewildering time, but at least we can become more aware of our own individual Selves.

I have spent decades racing through my life. I would cram as much activity into each day as I could, and that would result in my feeling I had done something. But now that such rushing about is not possible, it is not rewarded. I still want a sense of accomplishment and am an absolute lunatic about keeping my house tidy. I did not used to care that much, but if it is a mess, I feel a mess inside my head. Hence, I have learned to return things to a place I can find them again.

I am learning to savor relationships and not be as dependent on outside validation.

All in all, your advice has really helped. I have slowed down and multitask less often, although I still do my version of it. I am doing what I want to do but always somewhere inside have the sadness from realizing how devastating this past year has been for so many. So again, I thank you, Rumi, for expanding my ability to accept that which was certainly a jolt out of all our comfort zones.

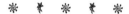

How is it that I am so enthralled by what I am learning? Is it because of the Qigong that I have been doing for twenty minutes almost every day for a year? Is it because of my listening to Marianne Williamson and doing Dr. Zach Bush's four-minute workout? Maybe my wearing my friend Miani's "prayer necklace" has helped? (She told me it would help with transformation.) How about my daily group meditation with Paula? Does that help? My dear friend Jessica simply tells me it is my slowing down. Slowing down is allowing me to hear these wonderful quotes and gather new awareness.

What have I become more aware of during these past months? The first thing is objectivity. Like holding a photo in my hand, I see things more as an observer. I am aware that I am letting more go to see what emerges.

I notice I am also not analyzing situations as much as I used to and no longer feel compelled to understand. I used to discuss behavior with friends and now I pretty much leave it be. It did not help me, and the further I let go, the more content I feel. Friendships are what have sustained me, and they continue to appear. I have no desire to alter them at all.

❁ ❋ ❁ ❋ ❁

"What would you do if you had a year to live?" Michael Lerner asked this in his journal on CaringBridge. I have been reading his journal on CaringBridge for over a year now because it nourishes me. I want to ponder this question a bit. My first response is that I would do nothing differently, but then I realize that perhaps that is not using my imagination, so I will stretch a bit.

What if I were able to travel to some warm place with year-round swimming in beautiful surroundings? I would do that if Monica would accompany me. I am still in pretty good health and enjoy each day, but I would swap locations for warmth and beauty.

So where am I now in my life? The age of seventy-seven means I am in a final section of my life, and I love that I feel unafraid of death. I am scared of suffering, but I hope that I will somehow be spared that.

This morning I am writing to see what I think, and it is really a pleasure. I am sitting in front of the fire, looking out at the snow, aware that the sun will soon be shining so I can go for a walk today.

The words that stick with me today come from when Sarah interviewed me on Halloween in 2003. She asked me, "What do you want your grandchildren to know?"

I got tears in my eyes and said, "Just to be kind." So, that is the bottom line for me, and I suppose I can now say that we *can* choose how we behave.

This reminds me of teaching four of my grandchildren when they were very young to dance the "Anger Dance." We were outdoors, and I was so clear on the importance of having them see that they were now old enough to choose to *not* have a temper tantrum. I felt the teaching moment worked that day, but who knows? Now I cannot get them to answer a text these days, so I feel left with uncertainty.

Do I actually know *anything* with certainty? Honestly, I am not sure! I wonder a lot about how a person can change their behavior, their character, or their personality. Can they actually alter their inner lives at all? My answer this morning is yes, and my reason is that I know I am remarkably more content than I was as a young person. Somehow my view of my Self has altered over the decades. I am choosing to write about this past year to focus on how I have thrived during a time that others have suffered such deep loss. You can dismiss this with "It's just that you are so privileged," but I think I have also consciously taken some steps that have altered my life.

I grew up on Park Avenue in NYC, went to private schools, did poorly in academic settings, and managed to still acquire two master's degrees. I did all that feeling stupid, and yet I chose to take on some hard programs and studied to earn two certificates in clinical pastoral education. I acquired these long education internships nineteen years apart, but that alone took guts. I now feel proud of having written long "verbatims" (reports of conversations with patients). These were difficult and demanded a lot of hard work, but I did them and am proud of taking on such a tough task.

I finally feel as though I can talk about my life in a way that will be a description of one woman's successful struggle to feel better. She now finally feels she is a worthwhile human being.

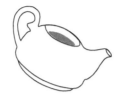

Conclusion

It is May of 2022, and my skin is on fire. I have wicked itching on my face, neck, and body where red splotches are, and I have had several nights of horrendous discomfort and scratching. Last night I got up at 3:00 a.m. to put on an eczema treatment that is in my freezer. The recipe comes from a friend in Scotland, and I put the two ingredients together over a month ago. It involved mixing Mānukora honey with my own urine, soaking cotton pads in it, and placing the pads in the freezer.

I include these details to show how intense the itching is so that you understand the level of my desperation. Last night it felt good to have the cold against my skin, and the itching did lessen, so I was able to go back to sleep for two hours. This morning, however, I am just as miserable with the itching and burning as I was yesterday.

Why do I believe that this is a necessary step in my healing process? I think the emotions I have repressed for decades are finally coming to the surface. I am no longer numb. They are finally being released.

I have been longing to be touched and I did not even know it. For the past month I have been having a passionate love affair with a man who is becoming the love of my life. He is eighty and I will soon be seventy-nine. I have never had anything that even comes close to these feelings and am able to feel dimensions of tenderness I never knew existed. I believe this may be why my body is in such a dramatic outburst. I am convinced this is my body and mind weeping. This love that I am feeling for the first time is opening wounds. I need to weep. Three marriages and I have never known this joy. No wonder my skin is burning up, not to mention the global crises of war, shootings, and climate change. We all are weeping in our own ways.

But I know that this extreme and painful skin reaction will calm down. It is now June of 2022, and I have been to a dermatologist who told me I actually had an infection, on top of the eczema. He is treating it with pills and cortisone, and my skin has finally cleared up. This doctor even acknowledges that the outbreak probably is connected to long-repressed feelings. I can now trust my body to heal. It actually *has* healed, and it is such a relief to no longer be either itching or burning.

This morning I heard Wergin on the internet explaining how we need to ask for healing. I remember how he told me that when my skin has an outbreak it means it is on its way out.

How grateful I feel to have asked for help and to believe it is here now. This weeping is a necessary step. How can we not be in awe of nature? I love waking up each morning, as I have just done, and writing in my journal with my pot of tea. I am basking in the feelings of being loved and of loving.

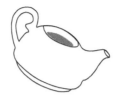

Reader Resources

My favorite learnings and books I recommend:

- *A New Earth: Awakening to Your Life's Purpose* by Eckhart Tolle
- *A Year of Miracles: Daily Devotions and Reflections* by Marianne Williamson
- *Atlas of the Heart* by Brené Brown
- *Barking to the Choir: The Power of Radical Kinship* by Gregory Boyle
- *Becoming* by Michelle Obama
- *Big Magic: Creative Living Beyond Fear* by Elizabeth Gilbert
- *Born a Crime: Stories from a South African Childhood* by Trevor Noah
- *Braving the Wilderness: The Quest for True Belonging and the Courage to Stand Alone* by Brené Brown

- *Caste: The Origins of Our Discontents* by Isabel Wilkerson
- *Dare to Lead: Brave Work. Tough Conversations. Whole Hearts.* by Brené Brown
- *Dying to Be Me: My Journey from Cancer, to Near Death, to True Healing* by Anita Moorjani
- *Emotional Inheritance: A Therapist, Her Patients, and the Legacy of Trauma* by Galit Atlas
- *Faith After Doubt: Why Your Beliefs Stopped Working and What to Do About It* by Brian D. McLaren
- *Flourish: A Visionary New Understanding of Happiness and Well-Being* by Martin E. P. Seligman
- *From What Is to What If: Unleashing the Power of Imagination to Create the Future We Want* by Rob Hopkins
- *In Pieces* by Sally Field
- *Inheritance: A Memoir of Genealogy, Paternity, and Love* by Dani Shapiro
- *Leaving Church: A Memoir of Faith* by Barbara Brown Taylor
- *Whole Brain Living: The Anatomy of Choice and the Four characters that Drive our Life* by Jill Bolte Taylor, Ph.D
- *My Beloved World* by Sonia Sotomayor
- *My Grandmother's Hands: Racialized Trauma and the Pathway to Mending Our Hearts and Bodies* by Resmaa Menakem

- *Nonviolent Communication: A Language of Life* by Marshall B. Rosenberg
- *Radical Acts of Love: Twenty Conversations to Inspire Hope at the End of Life* by Janie Brown
- *Radical Prayer: Love in Action* by Matthew Fox
- *Reaching Out: The Three Movements of the Spiritual Life* by Henri J. M. Nouwen
- *Rising Strong as a Spiritual Practice* by Brené Brown
- *Say What You Mean: A Mindful Approach to Nonviolent Communication* by Oren Jay Sofer
- *The Alcohol Experiment: A 30-day, Alcohol-Free Challenge to Interrupt Your Habits and Help You Take Control* by Annie Grace
- *The Art of Living: Peace and Freedom in the Here and Now* by Thích Nhất Hạnh
- *The Blue Sweater: Bridging the Gap Between Rich and Poor in an Interconnected World* by Jacqueline Novogratz
- *The Body Keeps the Score: Brain, Mind, and Body in the Healing of Trauma* by Bessel van der Kolk
- *The Book of Awakening: Having the Life You Want by Being Present to the Life You Have* by Mark Nepo
- *The Creative Habit* by Twyla Tharp
- *The Invisible World* by John O'Donohue
- *The Path Made Clear: Discovering Your Life's Direction and Purpose* by Oprah Winfrey

- *The Power of Giving Away Power: How the Best Leaders Learn to Let Go* by Matthew Barzun
- *The R.A.I.N. Meditation* by Tara Brach
- *The Seat of the Soul* by Gary Zukav
- *The Surrender Experiment: My Journey into Life's Perfection* by Michael A. Singer
- *Living Unthethered* by Michael A. Singer
- *The Turn Around Mom: How an Abuse and Addiction Survivor Stopped the Toxic Cycle for Her Family—and How You Can, Too!* by Carey Sipp
- *The Untethered Soul: The Journey Beyond Yourself* by Michael A. Singer
- *The Miracle of Mindfulness: A Manual on Meditation* by Thích Nhất Hạnh
- *Transforming Trauma: The Path to Hope and Healing* by James S. Gordon
- *Untamed* by Glennon Doyle
- *What Happened to You?: Conversations on Trauma, Resilience, and Healing* by Oprah Winfrey and Bruce D. Perry
- *You're Likely Not a Racist: Answers for Curious White People* by Teresa L. Reed

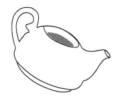

Bibliography

Acumen. "*Forbes* Names Jacqueline Novogratz as one of 100 Greatest Living Business Minds." September 19, 2017. https://acumen.org/blog/ forbes-names-jacqueline-novogratz-as-one-of-100- greatest-living-business-minds/.

Brown, Brené. *Atlas of The Heart: Mapping Meaningful Connection and the Language of Human Experience*. New York: Random House, 2021.

Oprah.com. "Golden Girl: Goldie Hawn on Happiness." January 26, 2011. https://www.oprah. com/oprahshow/goldie-hawn-on-happiness/all.

Powerful Non-Defensive Communication (PNDC). "What is PNDC?" Accessed June 3, 2022. https:// www.pndc.com/about/.

Rohr, Richard. *The Wisdom Pattern: Order, Disorder, Reorder*. Cincinnati: Franciscan Media, 2001.

Spangler, David A. "David's Desk 173 Climate Crisis." Lorian, October 1, 2021. https://lorian.org/community/2021/9/27/davids-desk-173-climate-crisis

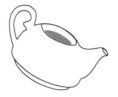

About the Author

Alexandra Cabot graduated from Columbia University and received Master's Degrees in Counseling and Psychology, and Social Work. Her life-long love of children led her to pursue working with and volunteering with families in educational and hospital settings. She has also worked as a hospice chaplain. She has four children and ten grandchildren. She currently resides in the Hudson River Valley.

You can reach the author at AuthorAlexandra Cabot@gmail.com

Lightning Source UK Ltd.
Milton Keynes UK
UKHW051236041022
409877UK00011BA/349/J